I0027080

HEALTHY SMOOTHIES

Vibrant and Wholesome Recipes for a Healthy You

BLEND AND SIP SAVOR THE RESULTS!

Dr. Kelafo Collie, M.D.

Shallaywa Collie, Ph.D

Majestic Priesthood Publications

Copyright ©2024 Dr. Kelafo Z. Collie, M.D., Shallaywa
Collie, Ph.D.
Healthy Smoothies

Vibrant and Wholesome Recipes for a Healthy You
Blend and Sip Savor the Results!

Recipe Book
ISBN 979-8-9906958-2-5
All rights reserved. No part of this book may be reproduced
or transmitted in any form or by any means without written
permission.
www.kelafozcollie.com
www.shallaywa.com
Published by:
Majestic Priesthood Publication,
Freeport, Grand Bahama, Bahamas.
Email: mpppublications@gmail.com
1-242-727-2137

Printed in the United States of America

Table of Contents

BONUS Smoothie Recipes

Introduction

Welcome to "Sip to Health: Nourishing Smoothies for Every Need," a recipe book dedicated to enhancing your well-being through the simple, delightful act of blending. In these pages, you'll discover a collection of smoothie recipes meticulously crafted to cater to specific health goals— whether you're managing diabetes, seeking gut-friendly options, aiming to shed weight, or focusing on enhancing your longevity.

Each recipe in this book is more than just a blend of ingredients; it's a fusion of science and nature, designed to deliver targeted health benefits without compromising on taste. The ingredients are chosen for their nutrient density, health-promoting properties, and their ability to work in harmony to nourish your body at a cellular level. From the antioxidant-rich berries and omega-packed seeds to the invigorating spices and greens, each smoothie is a step towards better health.

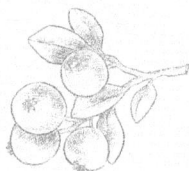

DIABETIC-FRIENDLY SIPS

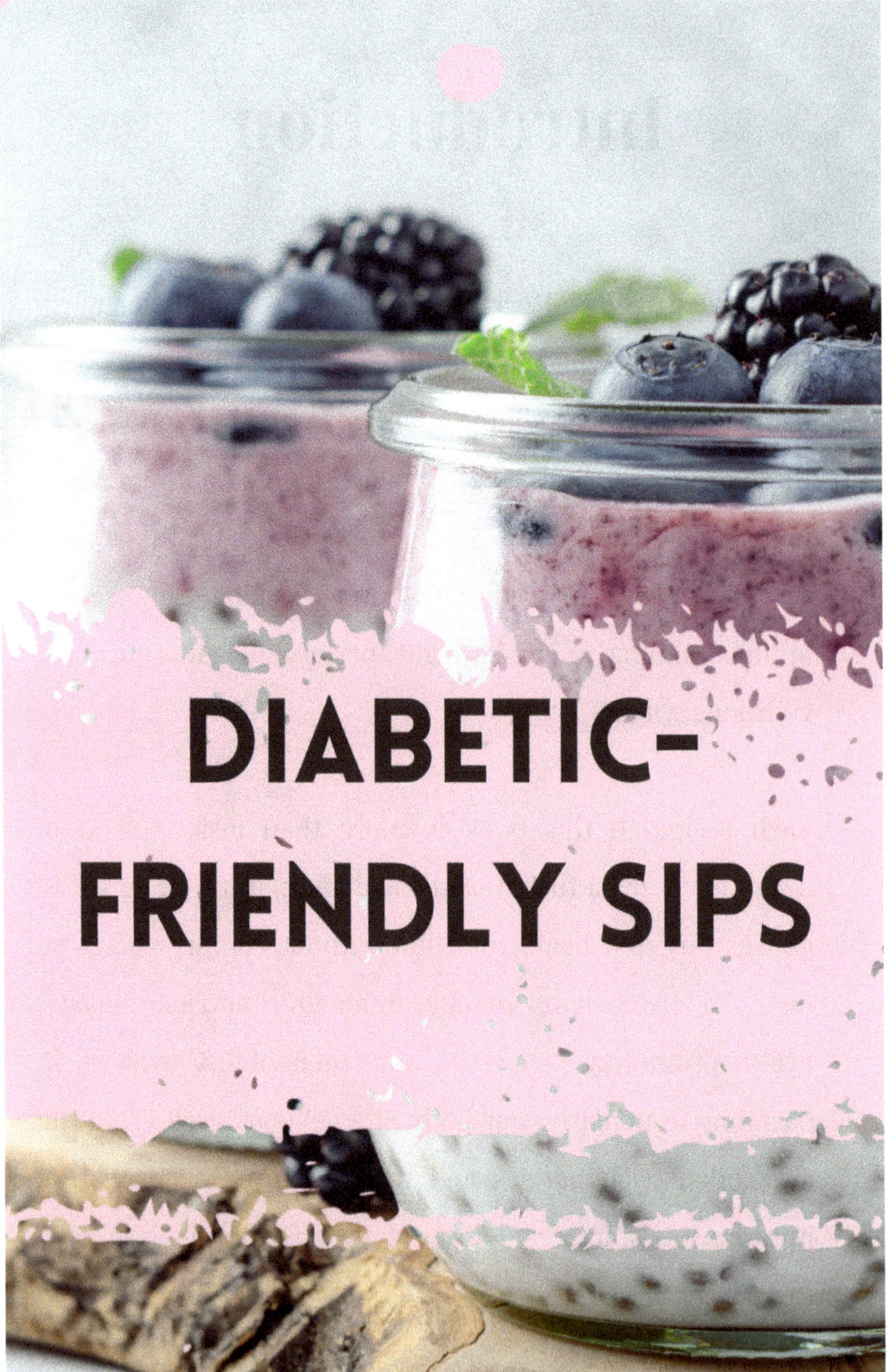

BERRY ALMOND SMOOTHIE

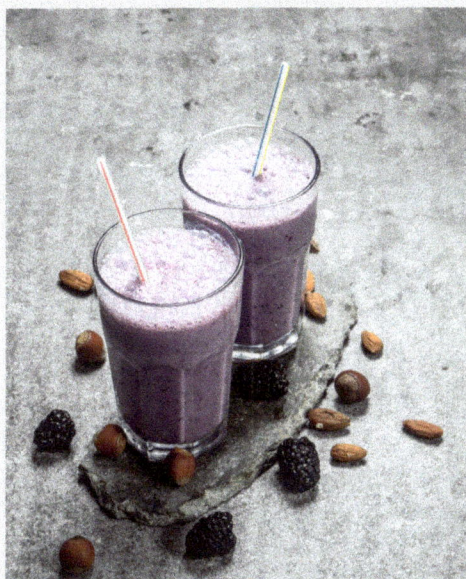

INGREDIENTS

- 1 cup mixed berries (strawberries, blueberries, raspberries), frozen
- 1 cup unsweetened almond milk
- 2 tbsp almond butter
- 1 tbsp chia seeds
- Stevia (optional, to taste)

DIRECTIONS

Place all the ingredients into a blender and blend until super smooth and creamy.
Serving: 1

NUTRITION FACTS

Calories	280kcal
Carbs	18g
Protein	8g
Fats	20g

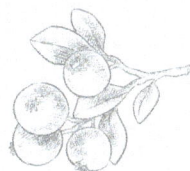

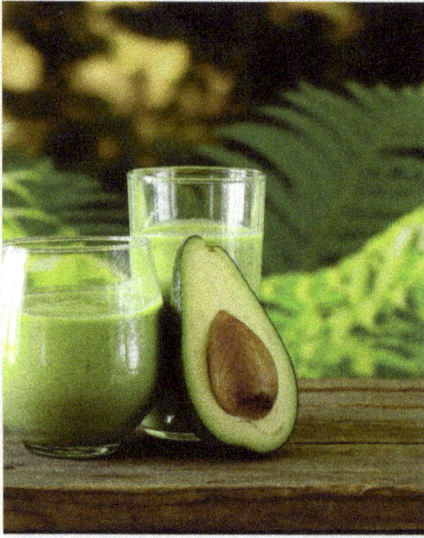

GREEN AVOCADO SMOOTHIE

INGREDIENTS

- 1/2 avocado
- 1 cup spinach leaves
- 1 small cucumber, chopped
- 1 tbsp ground flaxseeds
- 1 cup coconut water

DIRECTIONS

Place all the ingredients into a blender and blend until super smooth and creamy.
Serving: 1

NUTRITION FACTS

Calories	245kcal
Carbs	19g
Protein	4g
Fats	18g

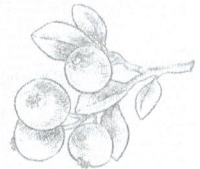

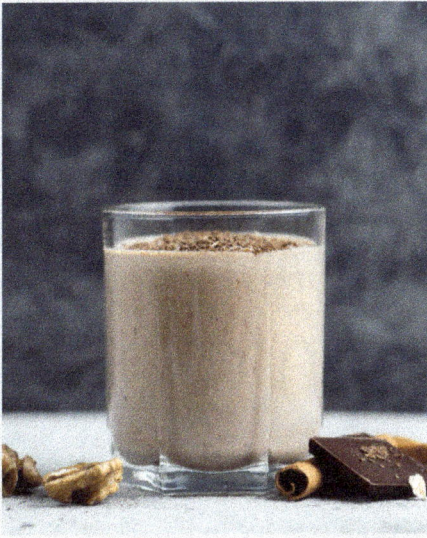

CINNAMON FLAX SMOOTHIE

INGREDIENTS

- 1/2 cup unsweetened Greek yogurt
- 2 tbsp ground flaxseed
- 1/4 tsp cinnamon
- 1/2 apple, peeled and chopped
- 1 cup water or unsweetened almond milk

DIRECTIONS

Place all the ingredients into a blender and blend until super smooth and creamy.

Serving: 1

NUTRITION FACTS

Calories	150kcal
Carbs	15g
Protein	9g
Fats	10g

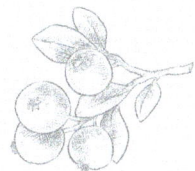

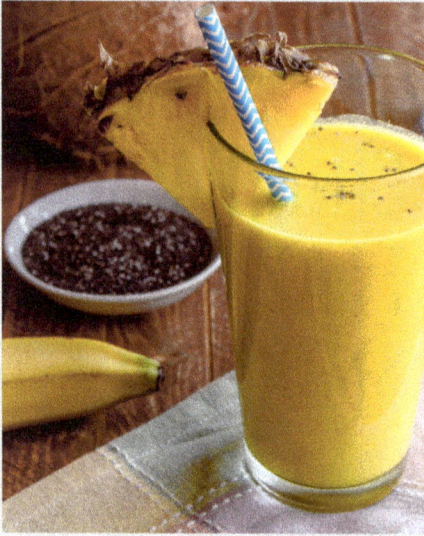

TROPICAL CHIA SMOOTHIE

INGREDIENTS

- 1/2 cup frozen mango chunks
- 1/2 banana
- 1 tbsp chia seeds
- 1 cup unsweetened coconut milk
- A squeeze of fresh lime juice

DIRECTIONS

Place all the ingredients into a blender and blend until super smooth and creamy.
Serving: 1

NUTRITION FACTS

Calories	210kcal
Carbs	29g
Protein	3g
Fats	11g

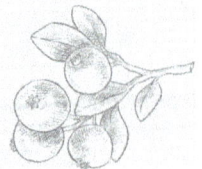

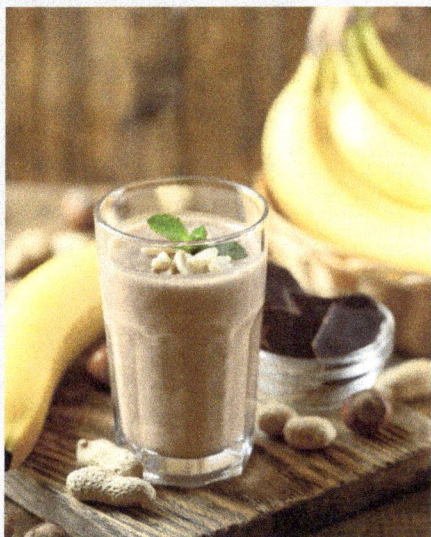

PEANUT BUTTER BANANA SMOOTHIE

INGREDIENTS

- 1/2 banana
- 2 tbsp natural peanut butter
- 1 cup unsweetened almond milk
- 1 scoop protein powder (vanilla or unflavored)

DIRECTIONS

Place all the ingredients into a blender and blend until super smooth and creamy.
Serving: 1

NUTRITION FACTS

Calories	340kcal
Carbs	21g
Protein	20g
Fats	22g

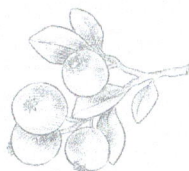

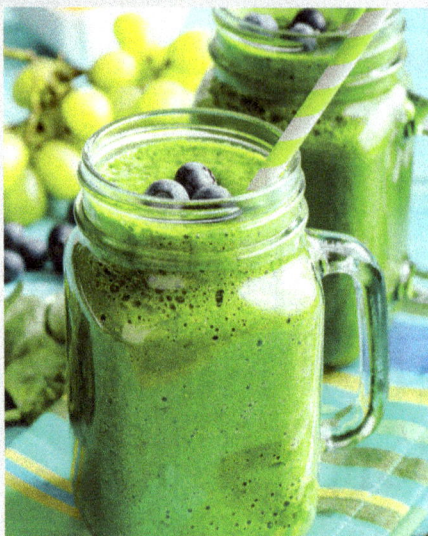

BERRY SPINACH SMOOTHIE

INGREDIENTS

- 1 cup spinach leaves
- 1/2 cup frozen blueberries
- 1 tbsp ground flaxseeds
- 1 cup unsweetened almond milk
- Stevia (optional, to taste)

DIRECTIONS

Place all the ingredients into a blender and blend until super smooth and creamy.

Serving: 1

NUTRITION FACTS

Calories	130kcal
Carbs	14g
Protein	3g
Fats	7g

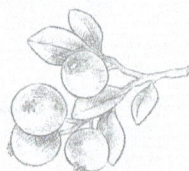

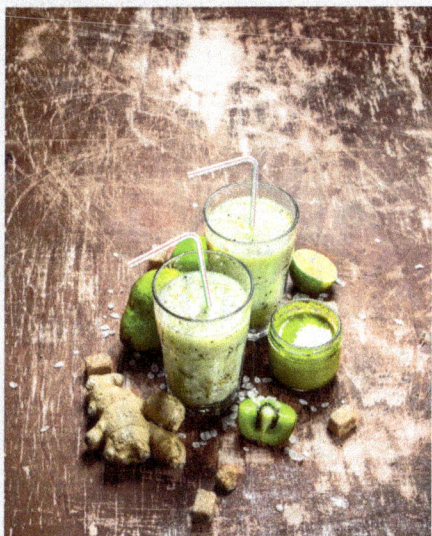

GINGER PEAR SMOOTHIE

INGREDIENTS

- 1/2 pear, cored and sliced
- 1/4 inch fresh ginger, peeled and minced
- 1/2 cup unsweetened Greek yogurt
- 1 tbsp hemp seeds
- 1 cup water

DIRECTIONS

Place all the ingredients into a blender and blend until super smooth and creamy.

Serving: 1

NUTRITION FACTS

Calories	170kcal
Carbs	18g
Protein	11g
Fats	6g

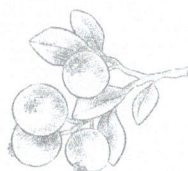

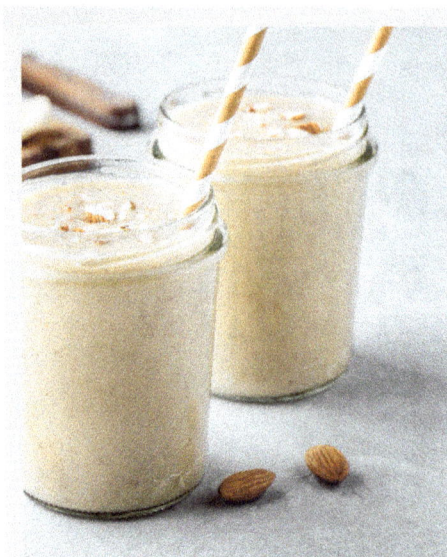

VANILLA PUMPKIN SMOOTHIE

INGREDIENTS

- 1/2 cup pumpkin puree (not pie filling)
- 1/2 tsp vanilla extract
- 1/4 tsp pumpkin pie spice
- 1 cup unsweetened almond milk
- 1 scoop protein powder (vanilla)

DIRECTIONS

Place all the ingredients into a blender and blend until super smooth and creamy.

Serving: 1

NUTRITION FACTS

Calories	180kcal
Carbs	10g
Protein	20g
Fats	3g

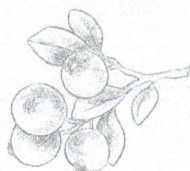

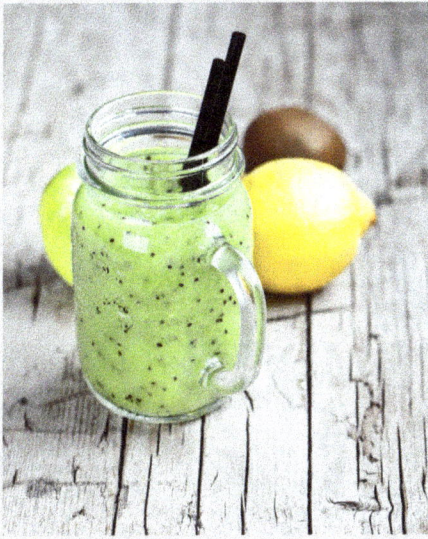

LEMON CHIA SMOOTHIE

INGREDIENTS

- Juice of 1 lemon
- 1 tbsp chia seeds
- 1/2 cucumber, sliced
- 1 cup water
- Stevia to taste
- Ice cubes (optional)

DIRECTIONS

Place all the ingredients into a blender and blend until super smooth and creamy.

Serving: 1

NUTRITION FACTS

Calories	70kcal
Carbs	9g
Protein	2g
Fats	3g

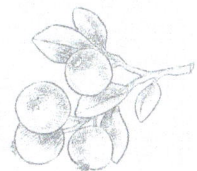

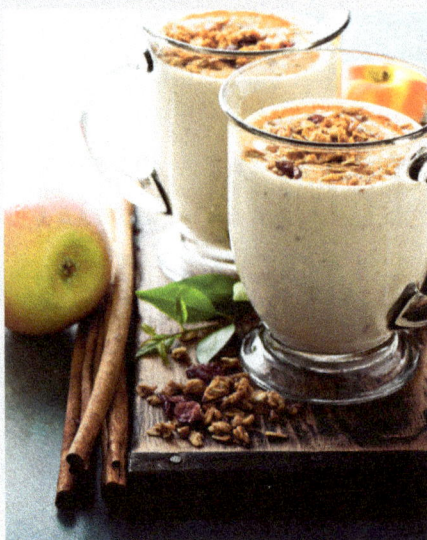

APPLE CINNAMON SMOOTHIE

INGREDIENTS

- 1/2 green apple, peeled and chopped
- 1/2 tsp ground cinnamon
- 1 tbsp almond butter
- 1 cup unsweetened almond milk
- Ice cubes (optional)

DIRECTIONS

Place all the ingredients into a blender and blend until super smooth and creamy.
Serving: 1

NUTRITION FACTS

Calories	160kcal
Carbs	18g
Protein	3g
Fats	9g

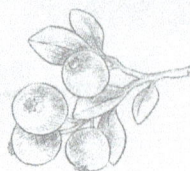

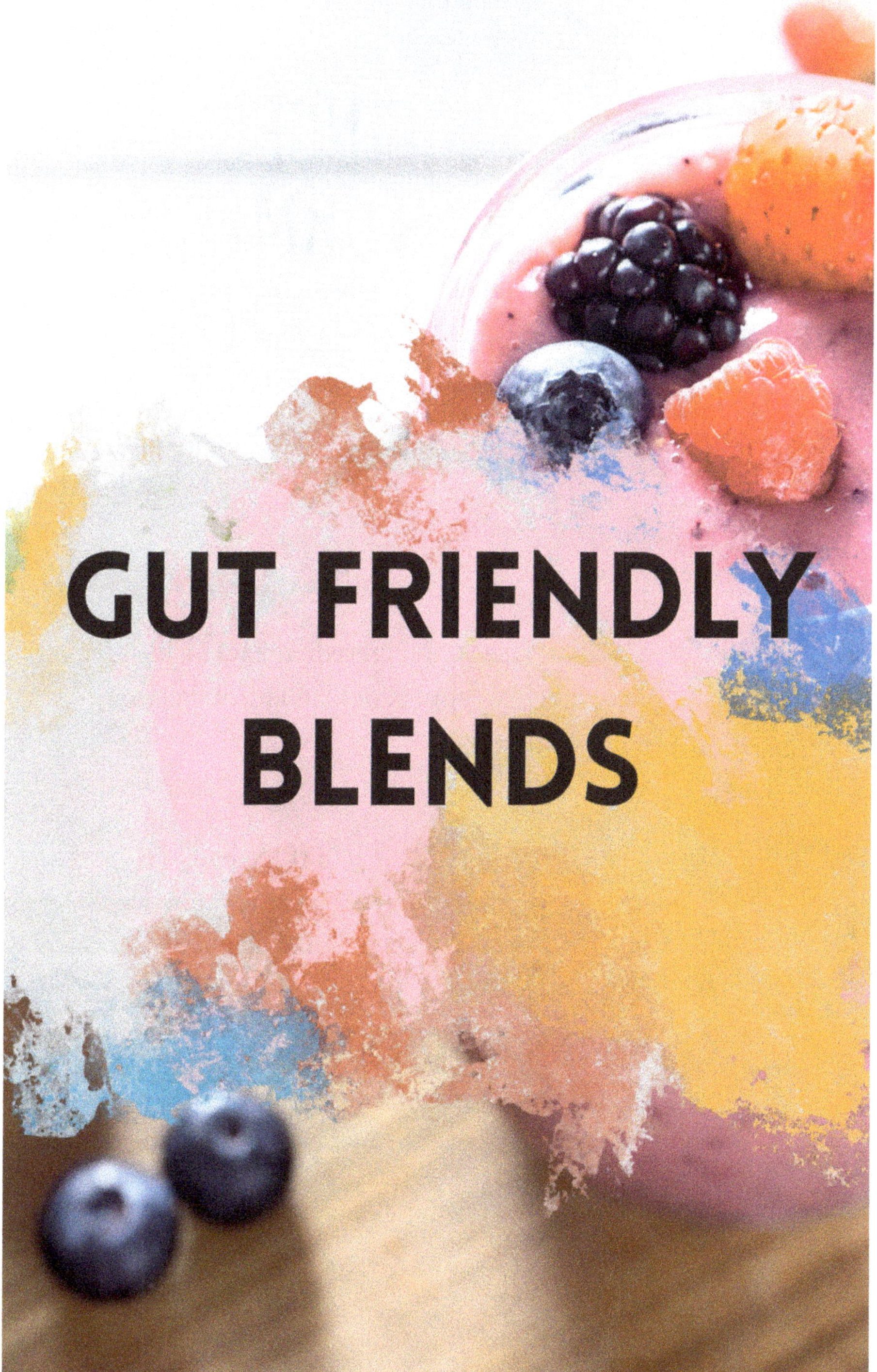

GUT FRIENDLY BLENDS

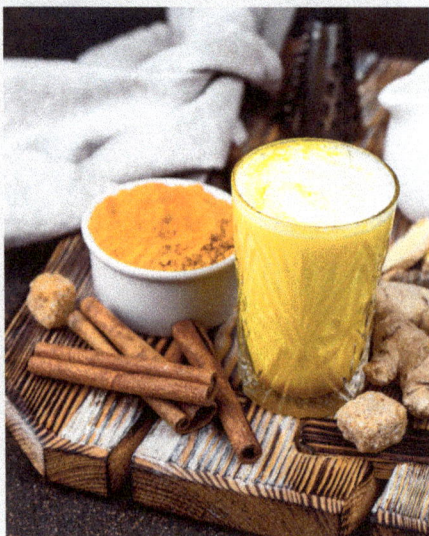

GINGER TURMERIC SMOOTHIE

INGREDIENTS

- 1 banana
- 1/2 inch fresh turmeric, peeled
- 1/2 inch fresh ginger, peeled
- 1 cup spinach
- 1 tbsp lemon juice
- 1 cup coconut water

DIRECTIONS

Place all the ingredients into a blender and blend until super smooth and creamy.

Serving: 1

NUTRITION FACTS

Calories	160kcal
Carbs	38g
Protein	2g
Fats	1g

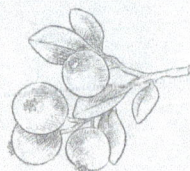

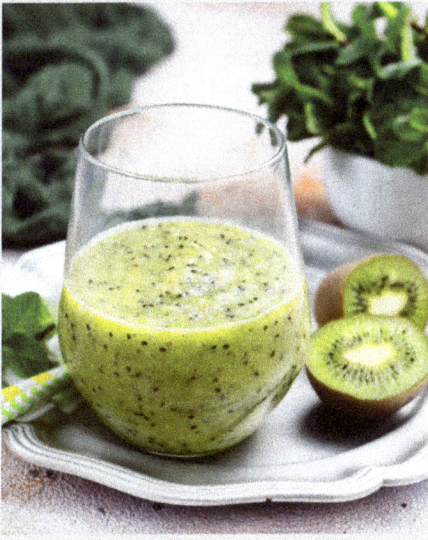

KIWI MINT SMOOTHIE

INGREDIENTS

- 2 kiwis, peeled and sliced
- 1/4 cup fresh mint leaves
- 1/2 cucumber, sliced
- 1 tbsp chia seeds
- 1 cup water

DIRECTIONS

Place all the ingredients into a blender and blend until super smooth and creamy.

Serving: 1

NUTRITION FACTS

Calories	150kcal
Carbs	30g
Protein	3g
Fats	4g

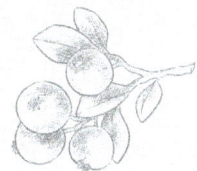

13

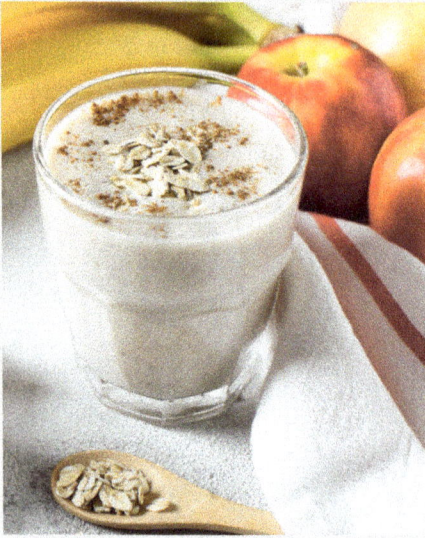

APPLE OAT SMOOTHIE

INGREDIENTS

- 1 apple, cored and sliced
- 1/4 cup rolled oats
- 1 tbsp almond butter
- 1/2 tsp cinnamon
- 1 cup unsweetened almond milk

DIRECTIONS

Place all the ingredients into a blender and blend until super smooth and creamy.

Serving: 1

NUTRITION FACTS

Calories	280kcal
Carbs	45g
Protein	6g
Fats	11g

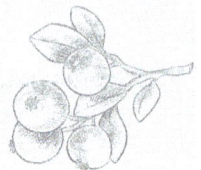

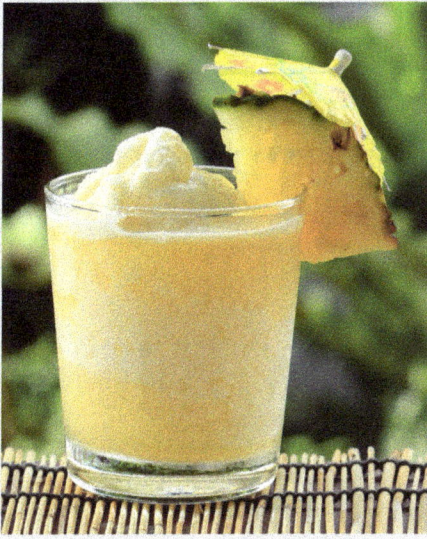

PINEAPPLE BASIL SMOOTHIE

INGREDIENTS

- 1 cup pineapple, chopped
- 1/4 cup basil leaves
- 1 tbsp flaxseed meal
- 1 cup coconut water

DIRECTIONS

Place all the ingredients into a blender and blend until super smooth and creamy.
Serving: 1

NUTRITION FACTS

Calories	140kcal
Carbs	33g
Protein	2g
Fats	1g

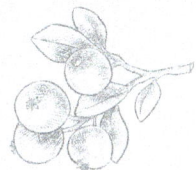

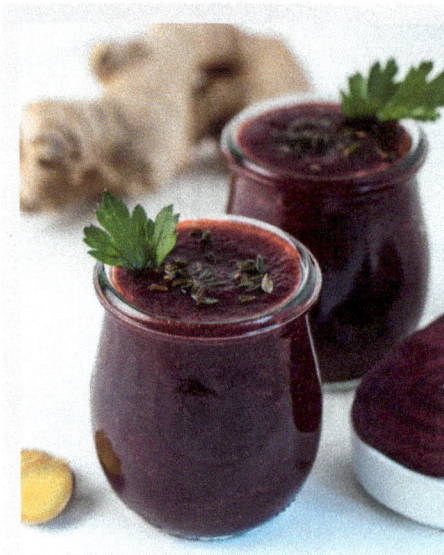

BEETROOT GINGER SMOOTHIE

INGREDIENTS

- 1 small beetroot, peeled and chopped
- 1/2 inch ginger, peeled
- 1 carrot, peeled and chopped
- 1 apple, cored and sliced
- 1 cup water

DIRECTIONS

Place all the ingredients into a blender and blend until super smooth and creamy.

Serving: 1

NUTRITION FACTS

Calories	120kcal
Carbs	30g
Protein	2g
Fats	0.5g

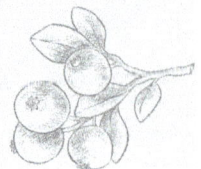

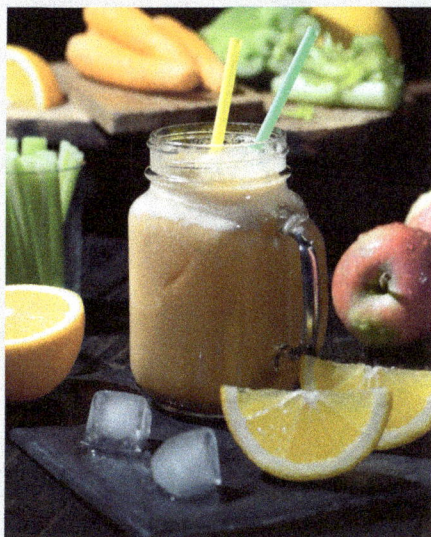

CARROT CELERY SMOOTHIE

INGREDIENTS

- 2 carrots, peeled and chopped
- 2 stalks celery, chopped
- 1/2 apple, cored and sliced
- 1 tbsp lemon juice
- 1 cup water

DIRECTIONS

Place all the ingredients into a blender and blend until super smooth and creamy.
Serving: 1

NUTRITION FACTS

Calories	95kcal
Carbs	22g
Protein	1g
Fats	0.5g

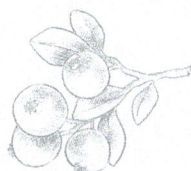

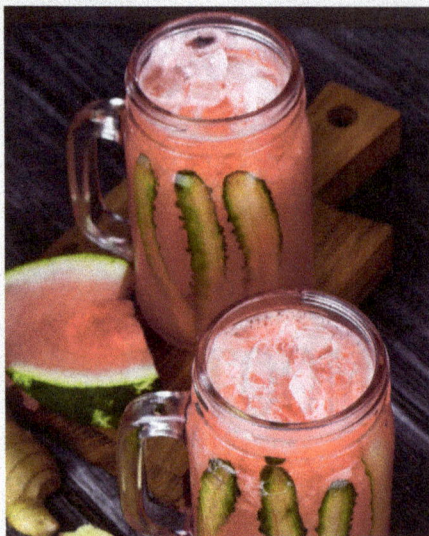

CUCUMBER MELON SMOOTHIE

INGREDIENTS

- 1 cup honeydew melon, chopped
- 1/2 cucumber, sliced
- 1/2 lime, juiced
- 1 tbsp mint leaves
- 1 cup water

DIRECTIONS

Place all the ingredients into a blender and blend until super smooth and creamy.

Serving: 1

NUTRITION FACTS

Calories	60kcal
Carbs	15g
Protein	1g
Fats	0.5g

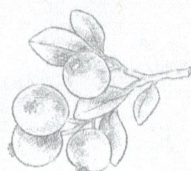

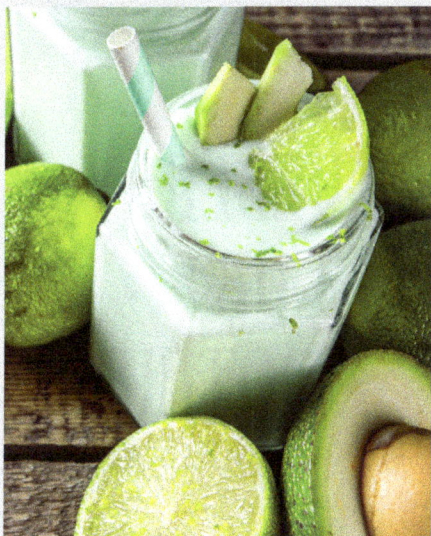

AVOCADO COCONUT SMOOTHIE

INGREDIENTS

- 1/2 avocado
- 1/2 cup coconut milk
- 1 tbsp lime juice
- 1/2 banana
- 1 cup spinach

DIRECTIONS

Place all the ingredients into a blender and blend until super smooth and creamy.

Serving: 1

NUTRITION FACTS

Calories	300kcal
Carbs	27g
Protein	4g
Fats	21g

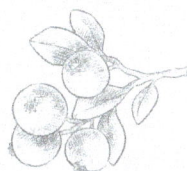

19

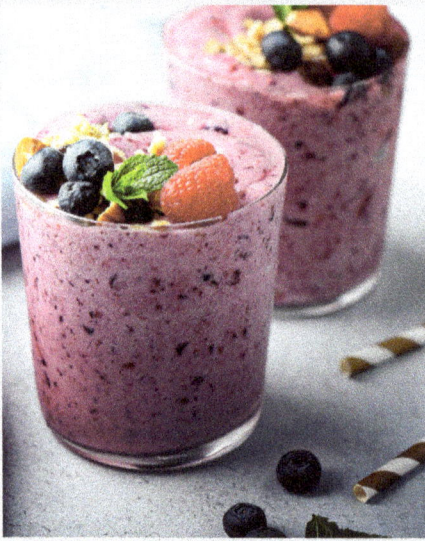

BLUEBERRY YOGURT SMOOTHIE

INGREDIENTS

- 1 cup blueberries, frozen
- 1/2 cup plain Greek yogurt
- 1 tbsp ground flaxseed
- 1 cup unsweetened almond milk

DIRECTIONS

Place all the ingredients into a blender and blend until super smooth and creamy.

Serving: 1

NUTRITION FACTS

Calories	190kcal
Carbs	28g
Protein	9g
Fats	6g

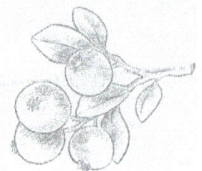

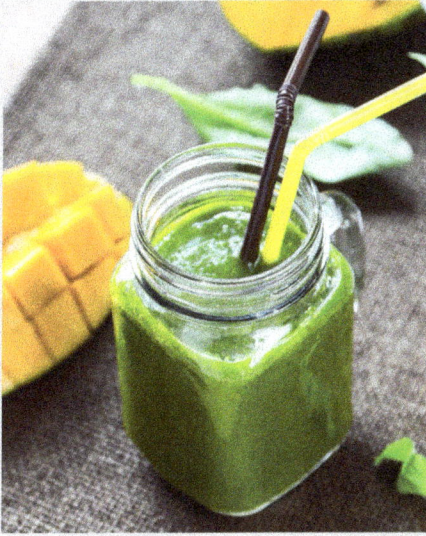

MANGO SPINACH SMOOTHIE

INGREDIENTS

- 1 cup mango, chopped
- 1 cup spinach leaves
- 1/2 banana
- 1 tbsp chia seeds
- 1 cup water

DIRECTIONS

Place all the ingredients into a blender and blend until super smooth and creamy.

Serving: 1

NUTRITION FACTS

Calories	200kcal
Carbs	45g
Protein	4g
Fats	3g

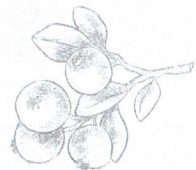

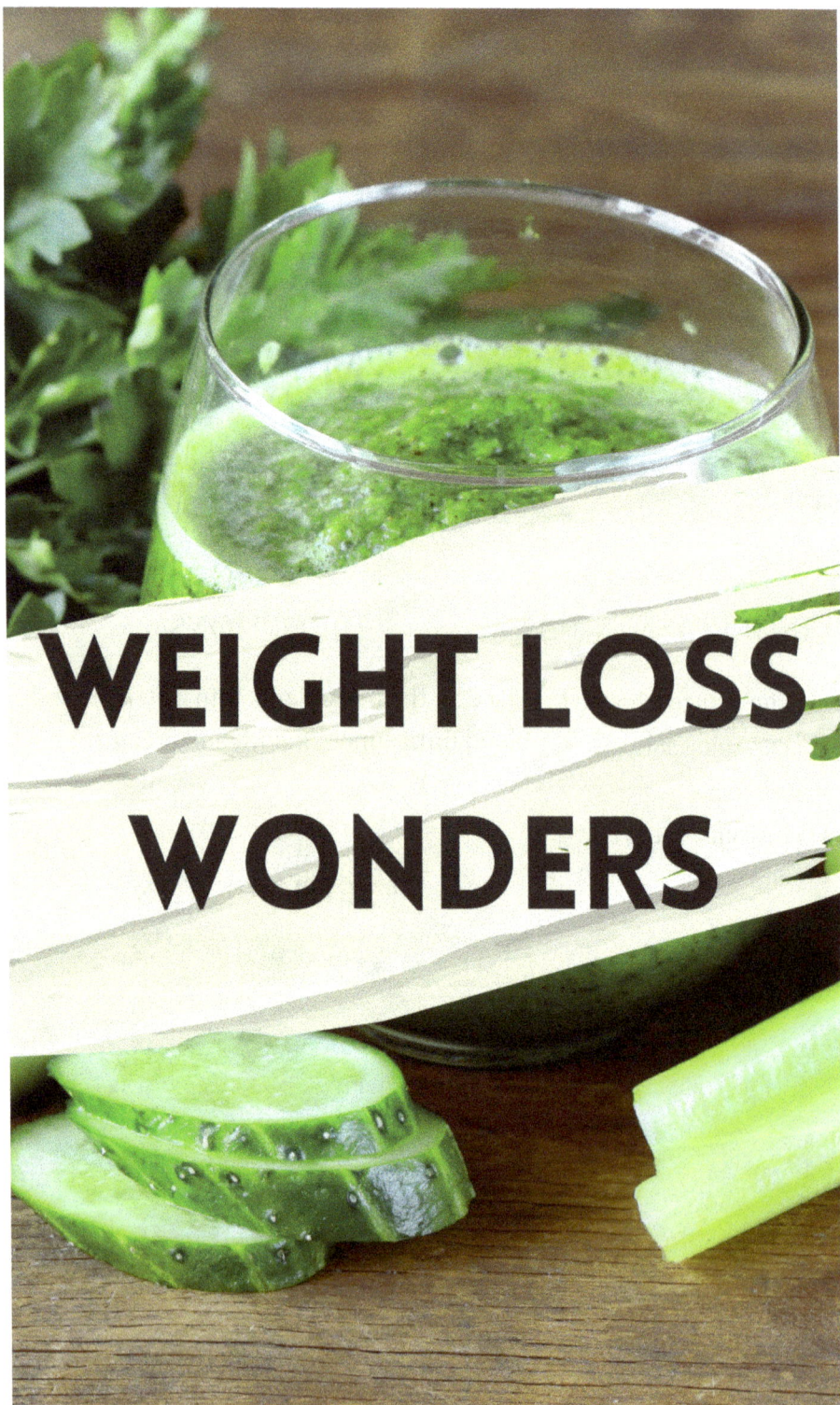

WEIGHT LOSS WONDERS

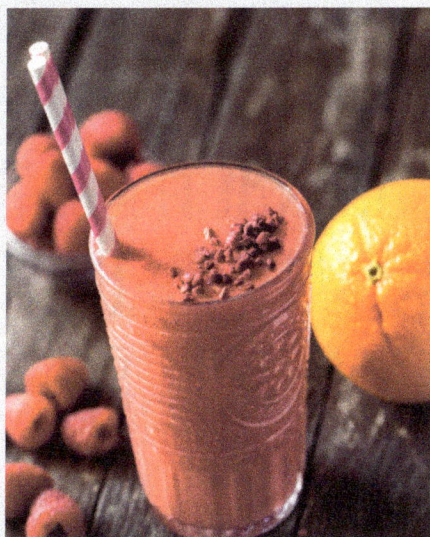

CITRUS BERRY SMOOTHIE

INGREDIENTS

- 1/2 grapefruit, peeled and seeded
- 1/2 cup strawberries, frozen
- 1/2 cup plain Greek yogurt
- 1 tbsp flaxseed meal
- Stevia to taste
- Water (as needed for desired consistency)

DIRECTIONS

Place all the ingredients into a blender and blend until super smooth and creamy.

Serving: 1

NUTRITION FACTS

Calories	150kcal
Carbs	18g
Protein	10g
Fats	4g

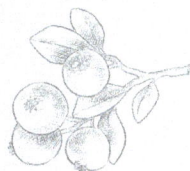

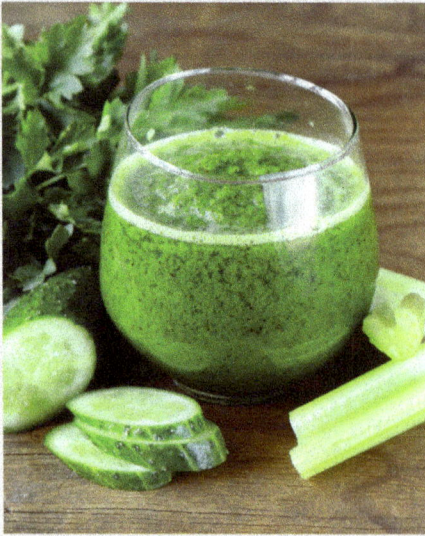

SPINACH CUCUMBER SMOOTHIE

INGREDIENTS

- 1 cup spinach leaves
- 1/2 cucumber, chopped
- 1/2 apple, cored and sliced
- 1 tbsp chia seeds
- 1 cup water

DIRECTIONS

Place all the ingredients into a blender and blend until super smooth and creamy.

Serving: 1

NUTRITION FACTS

Calories	100kcal
Carbs	17g
Protein	3g
Fats	3g

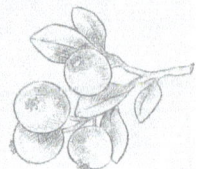

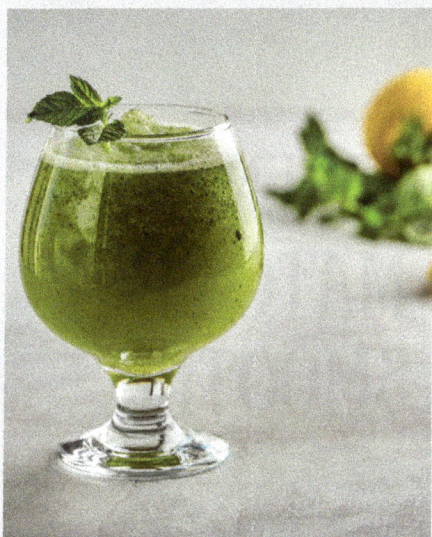

SPICY LEMONADE SMOOTHIE

INGREDIENTS

- 1 lemon, peeled and seeded
- 1/4 tsp cayenne pepper
- 1 tbsp honey (or substitute with a sweetener suitable for weight loss)
- 1 cup water

DIRECTIONS

Place all the ingredients into a blender and blend until super smooth and creamy.

Serving: 1

NUTRITION FACTS

Calories	70kcal
Carbs	19g
Protein	1g
Fats	0g

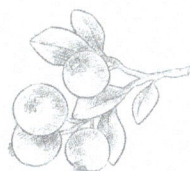

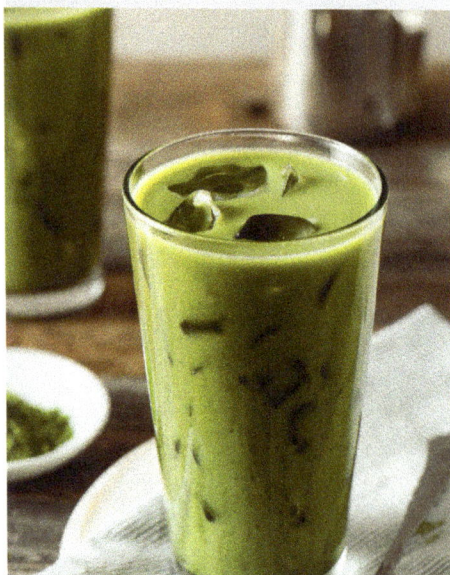

GREEN TEA MATCHA SMOOTHIE

INGREDIENTS

- 1 tsp matcha green tea powder
- 1/2 banana
- 1/2 cup spinach leaves
- 1 tbsp hemp seeds
- 1 cup unsweetened almond milk

DIRECTIONS

Place all the ingredients into a blender and blend until super smooth and creamy.
Serving: 1

NUTRITION FACTS

Calories	150kcal
Carbs	18g
Protein	6g
Fats	7g

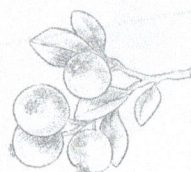

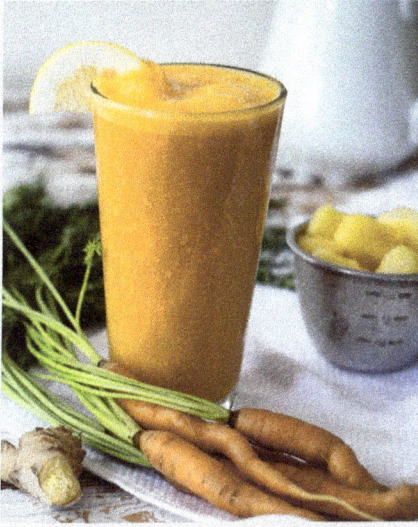

CARROT GINGER SMOOTHIE

INGREDIENTS

- 2 carrots, peeled and chopped
- 1/2 inch ginger, peeled
- 1 tbsp lemon juice
- 1 tbsp flaxseed meal
- 1 cup water

DIRECTIONS

Place all the ingredients into a blender and blend until super smooth and creamy.
Serving: 1

NUTRITION FACTS

Calories	95kcal
Carbs	17g
Protein	2g
Fats	3g

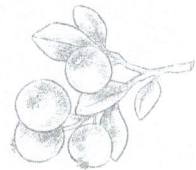

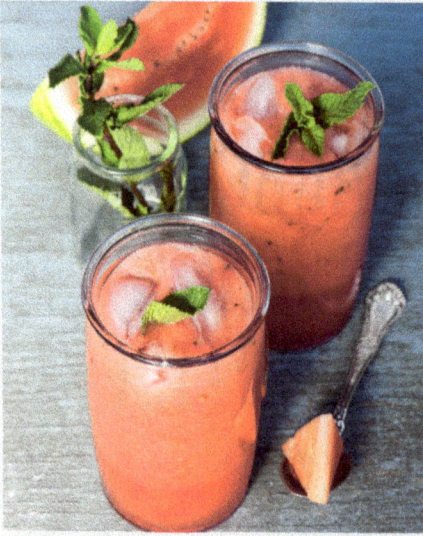

WATERMELON MINT SMOOTHIE

INGREDIENTS

- 2 cups watermelon, cubed
- 1/4 cup mint leaves
- 1/2 lime, juiced
- Water (as needed for desired consistency)

DIRECTIONS

Place all the ingredients into a blender and blend until super smooth and creamy.

Serving: 1

NUTRITION FACTS

Calories	90kcal
Carbs	22g
Protein	1g
Fats	0.5g

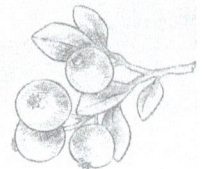

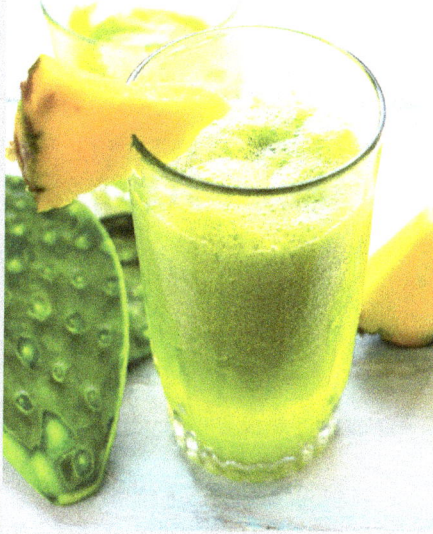

CELERY PINEAPPLE SMOOTHIE

INGREDIENTS

- 2 celery stalks, chopped
- 1 cup pineapple, chopped
- 1 tbsp chia seeds
- 1 cup water

DIRECTIONS

Place all the ingredients into a blender and blend until super smooth and creamy.

Serving: 1

NUTRITION FACTS

Calories	140kcal
Carbs	27g
Protein	2g
Fats	3g

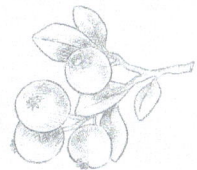

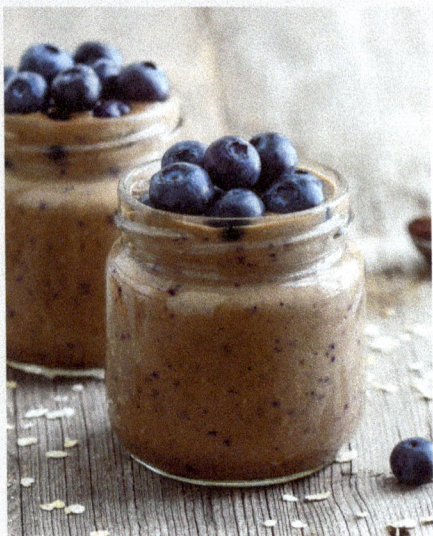

BLUEBERRY ALMOND SMOOTHIE

INGREDIENTS

- 1/2 cup blueberries, frozen
- 1 tbsp almond butter
- 1 tbsp ground flaxseed
- 1 cup unsweetened almond milk

DIRECTIONS

Place all the ingredients into a blender and blend until super smooth and creamy.

Serving: 1

NUTRITION FACTS

Calories	200kcal
Carbs	18g
Protein	5g
Fats	12g

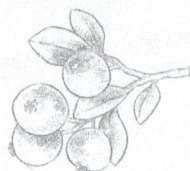

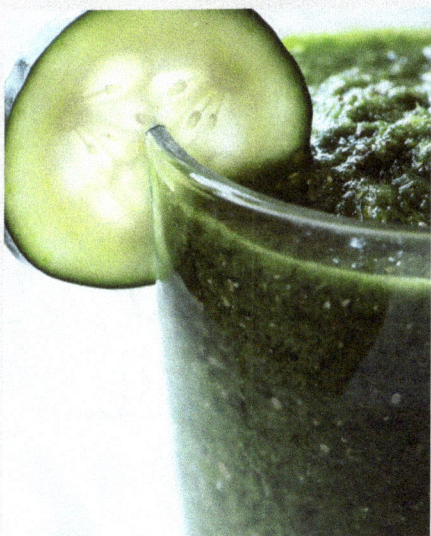

CUCUMBER KALE SMOOTHIE

INGREDIENTS

- 1/2 cucumber, chopped
- 1 cup kale, chopped
- 1 apple, cored and sliced
- 1 tbsp lemon juice
- 1 cup water

DIRECTIONS

Place all the ingredients into a blender and blend until super smooth and creamy.

Serving: 1

NUTRITION FACTS

Calories	120kcal
Carbs	28g
Protein	2g
Fats	0.5g

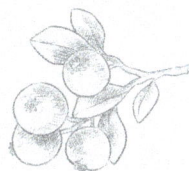

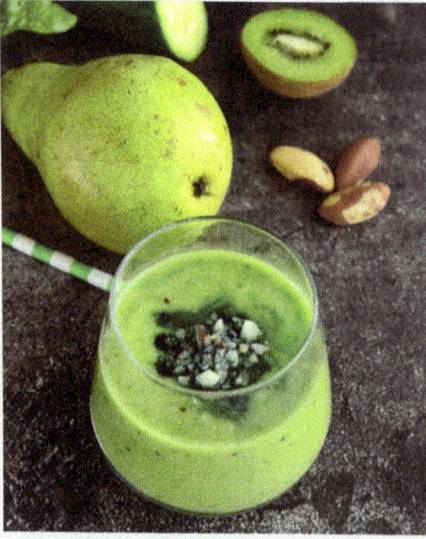

PEAR AVOCADO SMOOTHIE

INGREDIENTS

- 1 pear, cored and sliced
- 1/2 avocado
- 1 tbsp lemon juice
- 1 cup spinach leaves
- 1 cup water

DIRECTIONS

Place all the ingredients into a blender and blend until super smooth and creamy.
Serving: 1

NUTRITION FACTS

Calories	200kcal
Carbs	27g
Protein	3g
Fats	11g

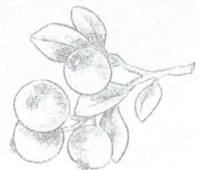

CANCER SUPPORT SIPS

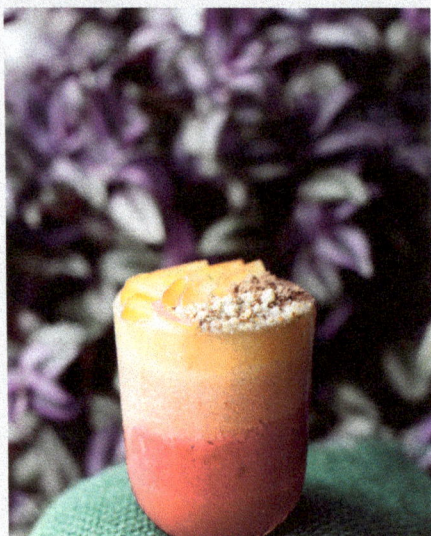

BERRY WALNUT SMOOTHIE

INGREDIENTS

- 1 cup mixed berries (blueberries, raspberries, blackberries), frozen
- 1 tbsp walnuts
- 1 cup spinach leaves
- 1 tbsp flaxseed meal
- 1 cup unsweetened almond milk

DIRECTIONS

Place all the ingredients into a blender and blend until super smooth and creamy.
Serving: 1

NUTRITION FACTS

Calories	180kcal
Carbs	20g
Protein	5g
Fats	10g

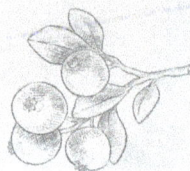

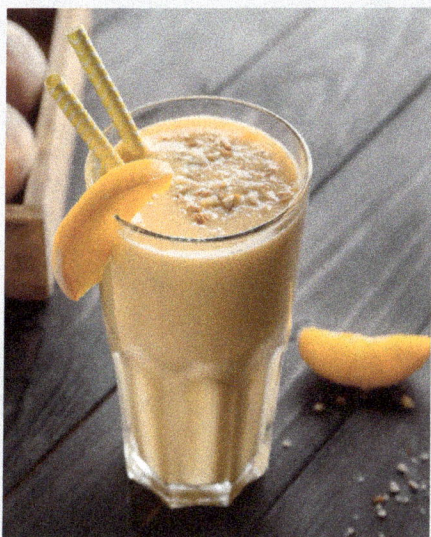

PEACH GINGER SMOOTHIE

INGREDIENTS

- 1 cup peaches, frozen
- 1/2 inch fresh ginger, peeled and minced
- 1/2 banana
- 1 tbsp chia seeds
- 1 cup coconut water

DIRECTIONS

Place all the ingredients into a blender and blend until super smooth and creamy.

Serving: 1

NUTRITION FACTS

Calories	150kcal
Carbs	35g
Protein	3g
Fats	2g

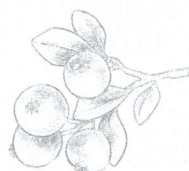

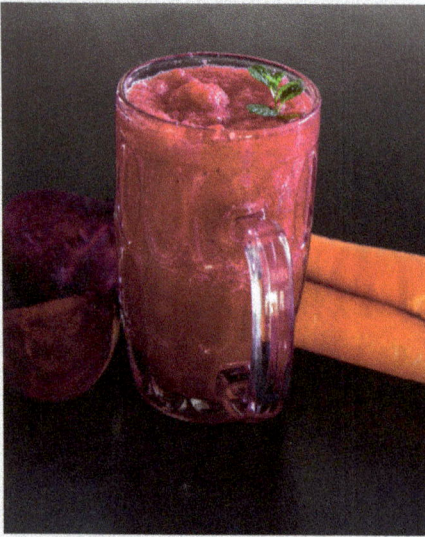

CARROT APPLE SMOOTHIE

INGREDIENTS

- 2 carrots, peeled and chopped
- 1 apple, cored and chopped
- 1 tbsp lemon juice
- 1 tsp turmeric
- 1 cup water

DIRECTIONS

Place all the ingredients into a blender and blend until super smooth and creamy.
Serving: 1

NUTRITION FACTS

Calories	120kcal
Carbs	30g
Protein	1g
Fats	1g

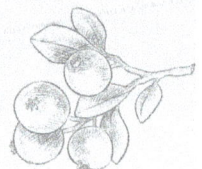

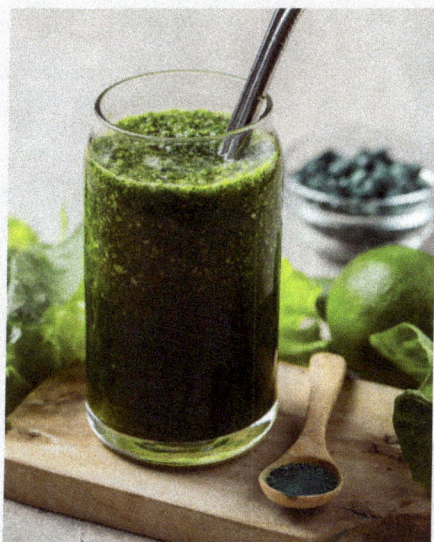

GREEN DETOX SMOOTHIE

INGREDIENTS

- 1 cup kale, stems removed
- 1/2 cup parsley leaves
- 1 celery stalk, chopped
- 1/2 green apple, cored and chopped
- 1 tbsp ground flaxseed
- 1 cup water

DIRECTIONS

Place all the ingredients into a blender and blend until super smooth and creamy.
Serving: 1

NUTRITION FACTS

Calories	100kcal
Carbs	20g
Protein	3g
Fats	3g

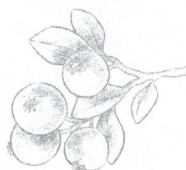

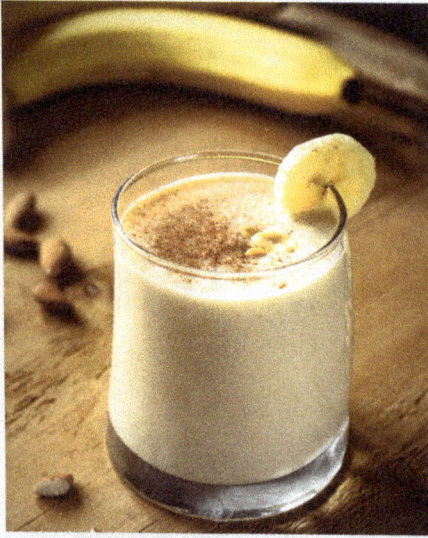

ALMOND BANANA SMOOTHIE

INGREDIENTS

- 1 banana
- 2 tbsp almond butter
- 1 tbsp cocoa powder (unsweetened)
- 1 cup unsweetened almond milk

DIRECTIONS

Place all the ingredients into a blender and blend until super smooth and creamy.

Serving: 1

NUTRITION FACTS

Calories	300kcal
Carbs	30g
Protein	8g
Fats	18g

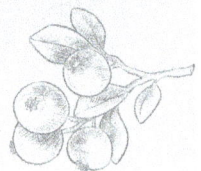

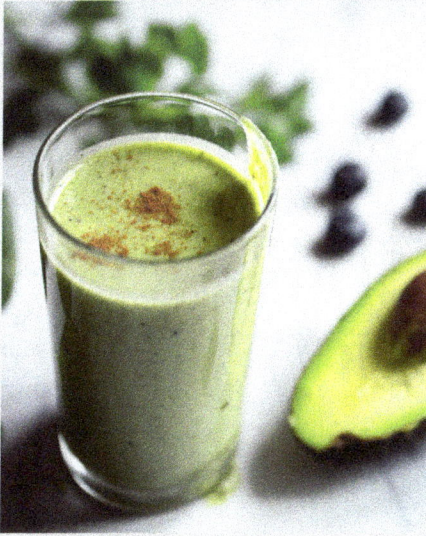

AVOCADO BERRY SMOOTHIE

INGREDIENTS

- 1/2 avocado
- 1/2 cup strawberries, frozen
- 1/2 cup blueberries, frozen
- 1 cup spinach leaves
- 1 cup water

DIRECTIONS

Place all the ingredients into a blender and blend until super smooth and creamy.

Serving: 1

NUTRITION FACTS

Calories	200kcal
Carbs	25g
Protein	3g
Fats	12g

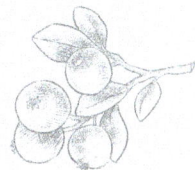

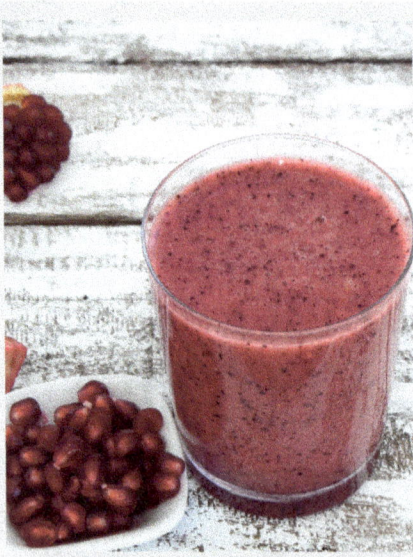

POMEGRANATE CITRUS SMOOTHIE

INGREDIENTS

- 1/2 cup pomegranate seeds
- 1 orange, peeled and seeded
- 1/2 banana
- 1 tbsp hemp seeds
- 1 cup water

DIRECTIONS

Place all the ingredients into a blender and blend until super smooth and creamy.

Serving: 1

NUTRITION FACTS

Calories	200kcal
Carbs	40g
Protein	5g
Fats	4g

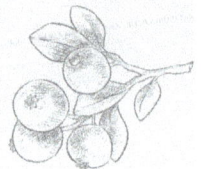

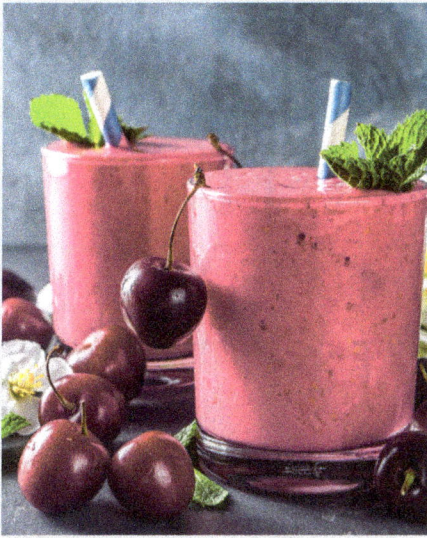

BEET AND BERRY SMOOTHIE

INGREDIENTS

- 1 small beet, peeled and chopped
- 1/2 cup raspberries, frozen
- 1 tbsp walnuts
- 1 tbsp chia seeds
- 1 cup coconut water

DIRECTIONS

Place all the ingredients into a blender and blend until super smooth and creamy.

Serving: 1

NUTRITION FACTS

Calories	180kcal
Carbs	28g
Protein	5g
Fats	6g

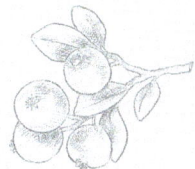

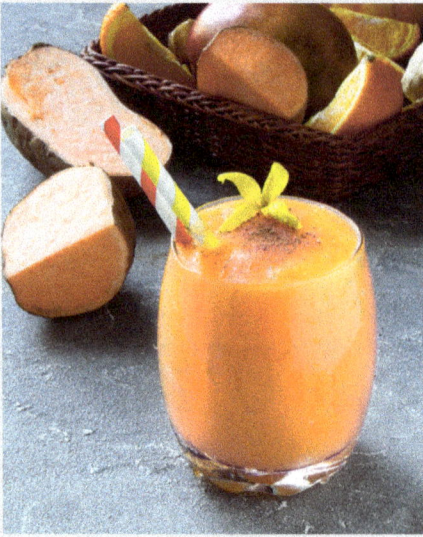

SWEET POTATO PIE SMOOTHIE

INGREDIENTS

- 1/2 cup sweet potato, cooked and cooled
- 1/4 tsp cinnamon
- 1/4 tsp nutmeg
- 1/2 banana
- 1 tbsp almond butter
- 1 cup unsweetened almond milk

DIRECTIONS

Place all the ingredients into a blender and blend until super smooth and creamy.

Serving: 1

NUTRITION FACTS

Calories	250kcal
Carbs	40g
Protein	5g
Fats	8g

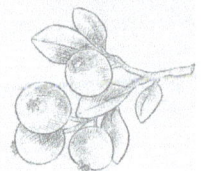

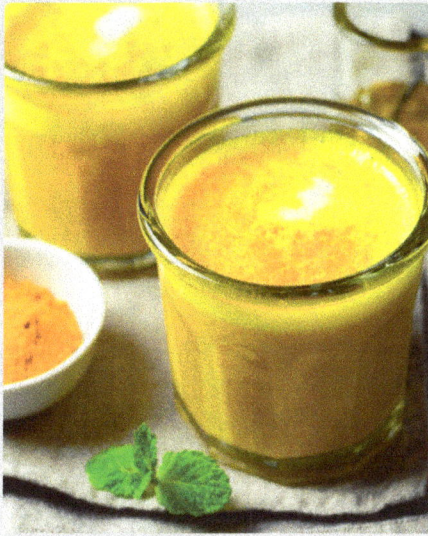

GOLDEN MILK SMOOTHIE

INGREDIENTS

- 1/2 banana
- 1/2 tsp turmeric powder
- 1/4 tsp cinnamon
- 1/2 tsp vanilla extract
- 1 tbsp almond butter
- 1 cup unsweetened almond milk

DIRECTIONS

Place all the ingredients into a blender and blend until super smooth and creamy.
Serving: 1

NUTRITION FACTS

Calories	200kcal
Carbs	22g
Protein	5g
Fats	11g

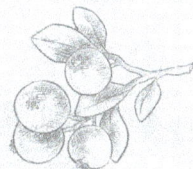

LONGEVITY ELIXIRS

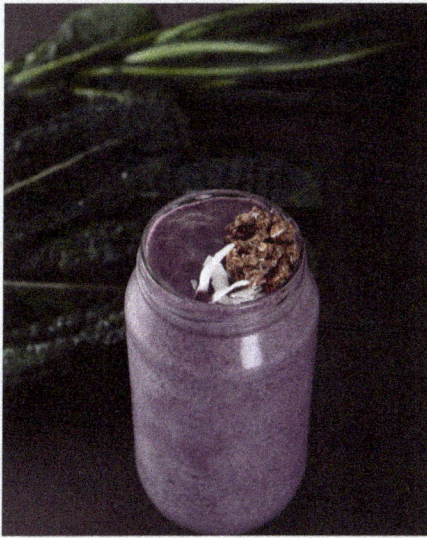

BLUEBERRY WALNUT SMOOTHIE

INGREDIENTS

- 1 cup blueberries, frozen
- 1 tbsp walnuts
- 1 tbsp flaxseed meal
- 1/2 cup spinach leaves
- 1 cup unsweetened almond milk

DIRECTIONS

Place all the ingredients into a blender and blend until super smooth and creamy.

Serving: 1

NUTRITION FACTS

Calories	180kcal
Carbs	20g
Protein	4g
Fats	10g

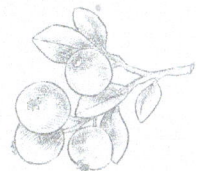

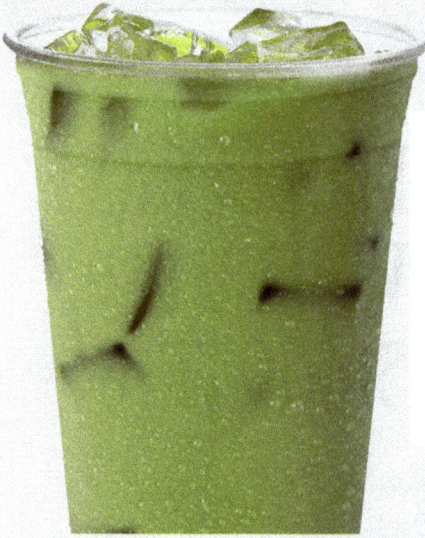

GREEN TEA INFUSION SMOOTHIE

INGREDIENTS

- 1 tsp matcha green tea powder
- 1/2 banana
- 1/2 cup mango, chopped
- 1 tbsp chia seeds
- 1 cup unsweetened almond milk

DIRECTIONS

Place all the ingredients into a blender and blend until super smooth and creamy.
Serving: 1

NUTRITION FACTS

Calories	180kcal
Carbs	28g
Protein	4g
Fats	6g

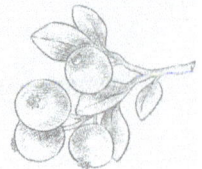

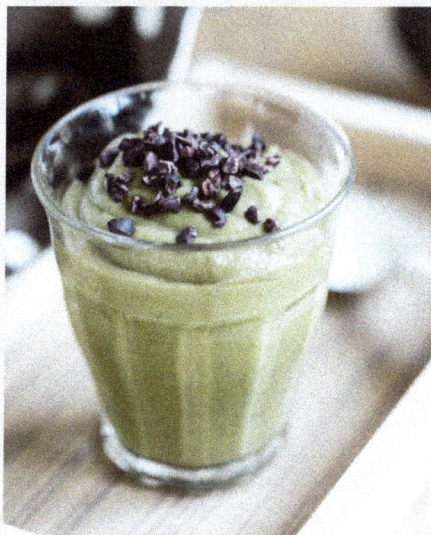

AVOCADO CACAO SMOOTHIE

INGREDIENTS

- 1/2 avocado
- 1 tbsp cacao powder
- 1 tbsp honey
- 1/2 banana
- 1 cup spinach leaves
- 1 cup unsweetened almond milk

DIRECTIONS

Place all the ingredients into a blender and blend until super smooth and creamy.

Serving: 1

NUTRITION FACTS

Calories	300kcal
Carbs	36g
Protein	5g
Fats	16g

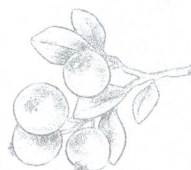

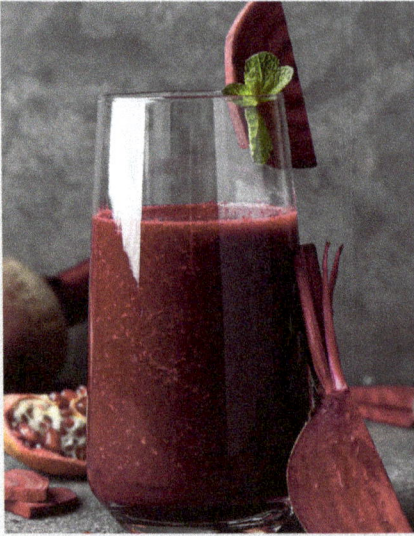

POMEGRANATE BEET SMOOTHIE

INGREDIENTS

- 1/2 cup pomegranate seeds
- 1 small beet, peeled and chopped
- 1/2 apple, cored and sliced
- 1 tbsp walnuts
- 1 cup water

DIRECTIONS

Place all the ingredients into a blender and blend until super smooth and creamy.

Serving: 1

NUTRITION FACTS

Calories	200kcal
Carbs	30g
Protein	4g
Fats	7g

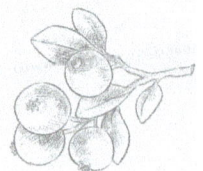

45

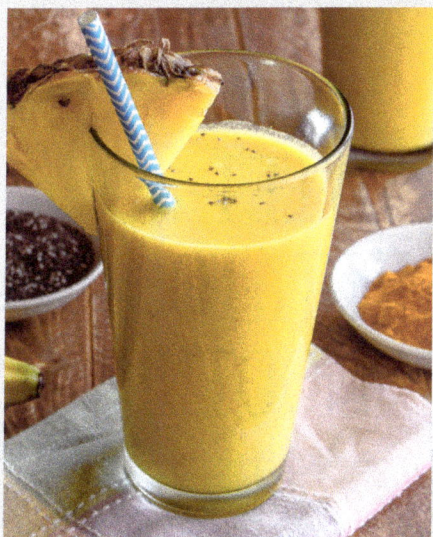

TURMERIC PINEAPPLE SMOOTHIE

INGREDIENTS

- 1 cup pineapple, chopped
- 1/2 tsp turmeric powder
- 1/2 inch ginger, peeled
- 1 tbsp flaxseed meal
- 1 cup coconut water

DIRECTIONS

Place all the ingredients into a blender and blend until super smooth and creamy.

Serving: 1

NUTRITION FACTS

Calories	180kcal
Carbs	40g
Protein	2g
Fats	2g

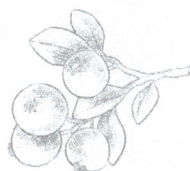

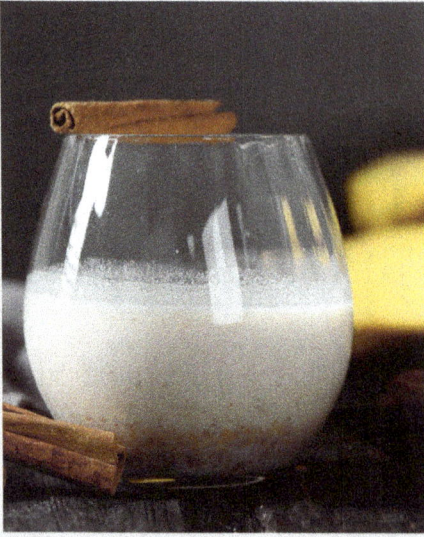

SWEET POTATO SMOOTHIE

INGREDIENTS

- 1/2 cup sweet potato, cooked and cooled
- 1/4 tsp cinnamon
- 1/2 banana
- 1 tbsp almond butter
- 1 cup unsweetened almond milk

DIRECTIONS

Place all the ingredients into a blender and blend until super smooth and creamy.
Serving: 1

NUTRITION FACTS

Calories	250kcal
Carbs	38g
Protein	5g
Fats	8g

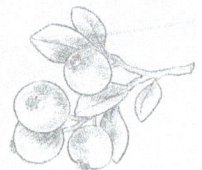

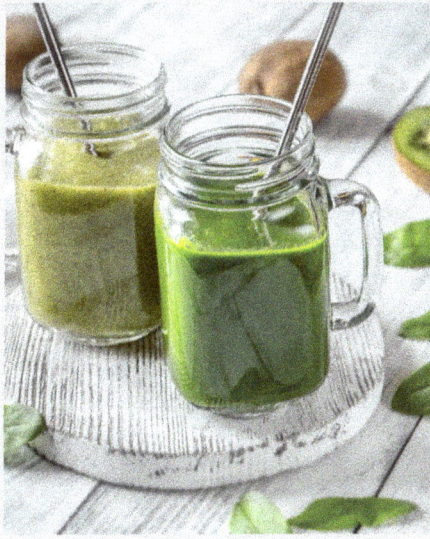

SPINACH AND KIWI SMOOTHIE

INGREDIENTS

- 1 cup spinach leaves
- 2 kiwis, peeled and sliced
- 1/2 cucumber, sliced
- 1 tbsp hemp seeds
- 1 cup water

DIRECTIONS

Place all the ingredients into a blender and blend until super smooth and creamy.

Serving: 1

NUTRITION FACTS

Calories	150kcal
Carbs	20g
Protein	6g
Fats	5g

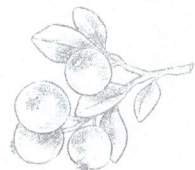

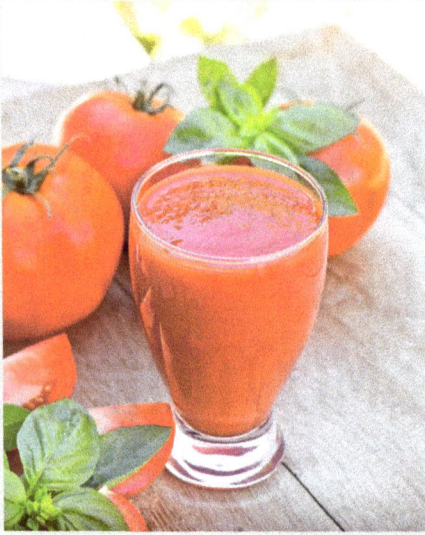

TOMATO BASIL SMOOTHIE

INGREDIENTS

- 1 cup tomatoes, chopped
- 1/4 cup fresh basil leaves
- 1/2 carrot, chopped
- 1 tbsp hemp seeds
- 1 cup water

DIRECTIONS

Place all the ingredients into a blender and blend until super smooth and creamy.

Serving: 1

NUTRITION FACTS

Calories	90kcal
Carbs	10g
Protein	4g
Fats	4g

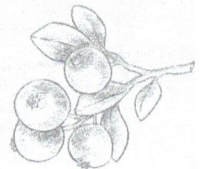

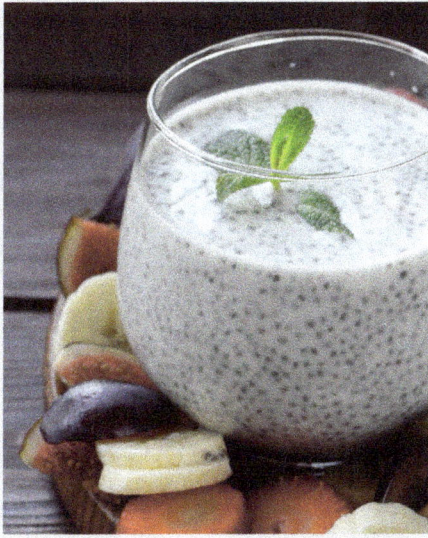

NUTTY OMEGA SMOOTHIE

INGREDIENTS

- 1 tbsp ground flaxseeds
- 1 tbsp walnuts
- 1/2 banana
- 1/2 cup blueberries, frozen
- 1 cup spinach leaves
- 1 cup unsweetened almond milk

DIRECTIONS

Place all the ingredients into a blender and blend until super smooth and creamy.
Serving: 1

NUTRITION FACTS

Calories	220kcal
Carbs	28g
Protein	5g
Fats	11g

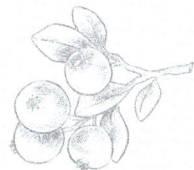

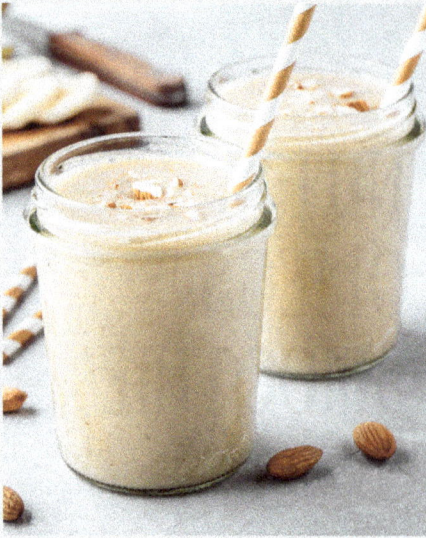

ALMOND AND DATE SMOOTHIE

INGREDIENTS

- 5 dates, pitted
- 2 tbsp almond butter
- 1/2 tsp vanilla extract
- 1 cup unsweetened almond milk
- Ice cubes (optional)

DIRECTIONS

Place all the ingredients into a blender and blend until super smooth and creamy.

Serving: 1

NUTRITION FACTS

Calories	320kcal
Carbs	50g
Protein	7g
Fats	13g

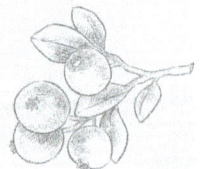

BONUS

SMOOTHIE

RECIPES

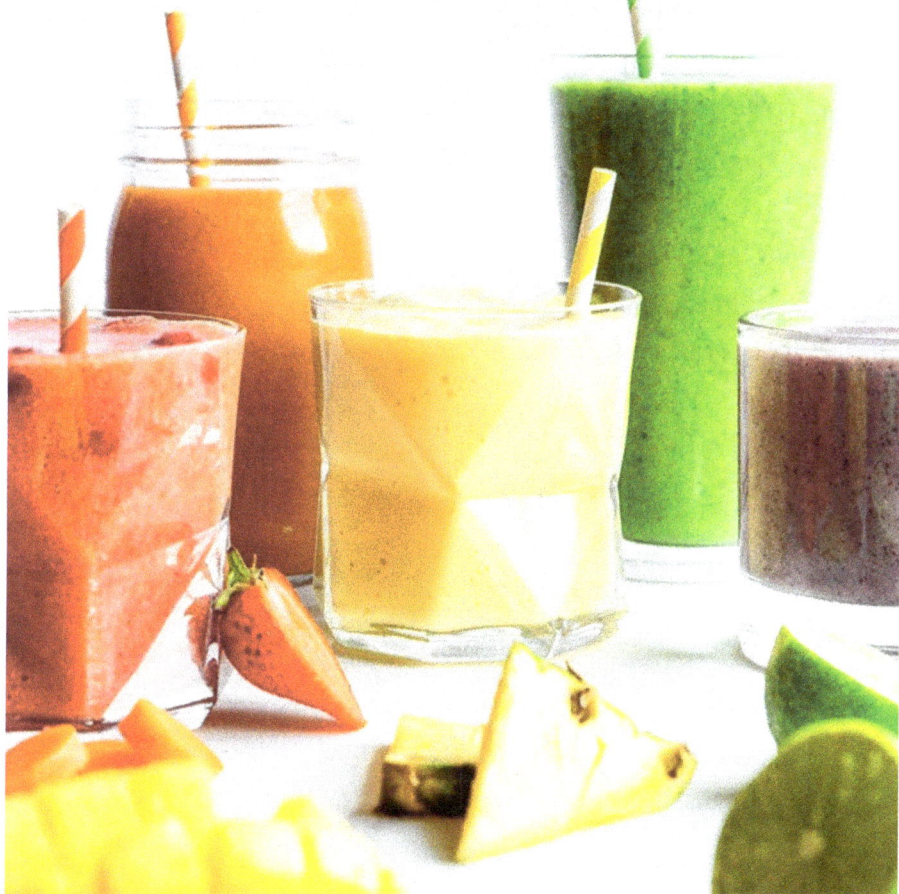

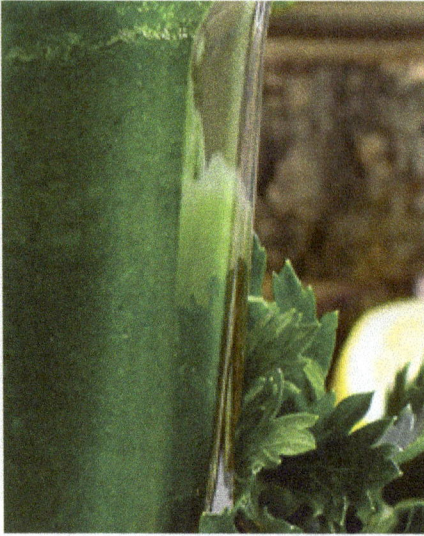

NOURISHING SMOOTHIE RECIPE

INGREDIENTS

- 1 cup vanilla almond milk
- 2 cups looselypacked kale
- 1 Granny Smith apple
- 1 organic lime, juiced
- 2 teaspoons raw honey

DIRECTIONS

Mix together all ingredients in the blender. Pulse for 30 seconds on low speed, adjust to high and pulse until smooth. Serve immediately.

NUTRITION FACTS

Calories	288.5kcal
Carbs	37g
Protein	3.7g
Fats	16.5g
Fiber	10.5g
Sugar	20g

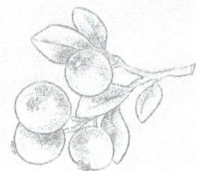

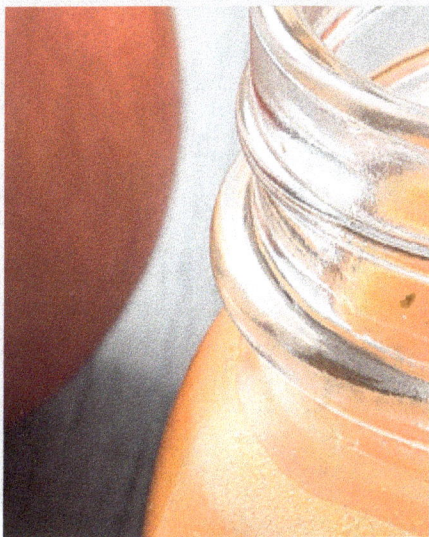

DETOX SMOOTHIE RECIPE

INGREDIENTS

- ½ cup orange juice
- 1 cup of coconut water (optional) 4 kernels of Brazil nuts
- 1 cup frozenpineapple chunks
- 1 cup looselypacked baby spinach 2 medium stalk of celery
- 1-inch piece lemongrass stalk 1 medium apple
-

DIRECTIONS

Mix together all ingredients in the blender. Pulse for 30 seconds on low speed, adjust to high and pulse until smooth. Serve immediately.

NUTRITION FACTS

Calories	281kcal
Carbs	58g
Protein	4.2g
Fats	7.5g
Fiber	6g
Sugar	34g

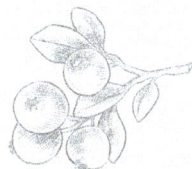

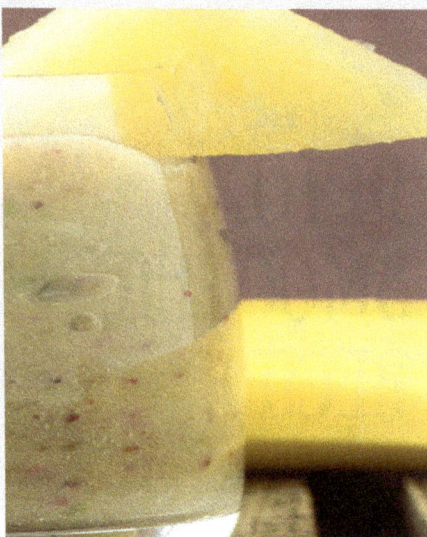

WEIGHT LOSS SMOOTHIE RECIPE

INGREDIENTS

- 1 cup unsweetened almond milk
- ½ cup fresh pineapple juice 1 ripe banana
- 1 cup guava, seeded
- 1 cup diced frozen watermelon 2 cups packed baby spinach
- 1 tablespoon of raw honey

DIRECTIONS

Mix together all ingredients in the blender. Pulse for 30 seconds on low speed, adjust to high and pulse until smooth. Serve immediately.

NUTRITION FACTS

Calories	185.5kcal
Carbs	41.5g
Protein	3.7g
Fats	2.2g
Fiber	4.1g
Sugar	29.5g

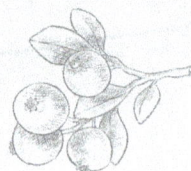

ANTI-AGING SMOOTHIE RECIPE

INGREDIENTS

- 1 cup unsweetened almond milk
- ½ cup Greekyogurt 2 kiwis
- 1 avocado
- 1 cup frozen blueberry
- ½ cup pomegranate arils
- 1 tablespoon maplesyrup (optional
-

DIRECTIONS

Mix together all ingredients in the blender. Pulse for 30 seconds on low speed, adjust to high and pulse until smooth. Serve immediately.

NUTRITION FACTS

Calories	298.5kcal
Carbs	37.5g
Protein	4.3g
Fats	17g
Fiber	13.5g
Sugar	29g

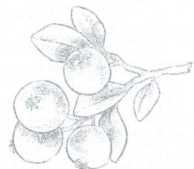

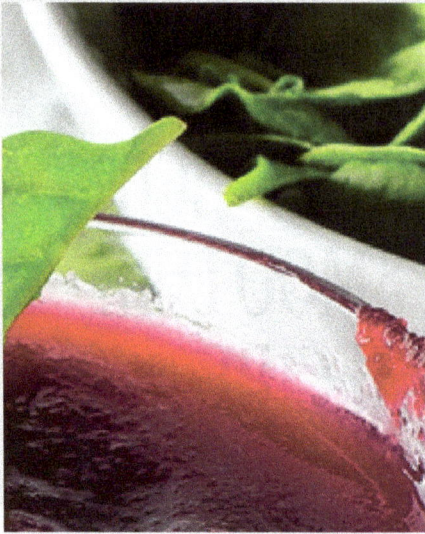

IMMUNE-BOOSTING SMOOTHIE

INGREDIENTS

- ½ cup cranberry juice 1 cup Greek yogurt
- 1 orange, segmented
- 1 grapefruit, segmented 1 cup frozen blueberries
- ¼ cup dried Goji berries
- 2 cups loosely packed kale

DIRECTIONS

Mix together all ingredients in the blender. Pulse for 30 seconds on low speed, adjust to high and pulse until smooth. Serve immediately.

NUTRITION FACTS

Calories	240kcal
Carbs	45.5g
Protein	15.5g
Fats	1.1g
Fiber	5.5g
Sugar	25.5g

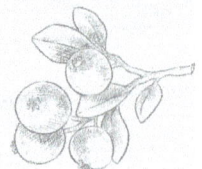

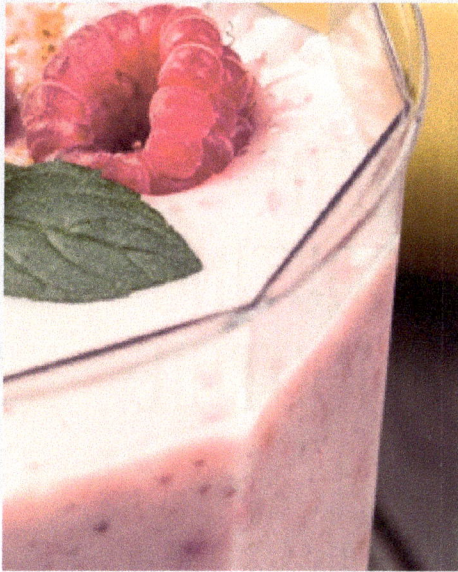

ENERGIZING SMOOTHIE RECIPE

INGREDIENTS

- 2 cups frozen raspberries 1 cup vanilla almond milk
- 2 tablespoons almondbutter 1 ripe banana
- 2 cups looselypacked kale 1 orange, segmented
- 1 teaspoon raw honey

DIRECTIONS

Mix together all ingredients in the blender. Pulse for 30 seconds on low speed, adjust to high and pulse until smooth. Serve immediately.

NUTRITION FACTS

Calories	27kcal
Carbs	42g
Protein	7.5g
Fats	11.5g
Fiber	13.5g
Sugar	20g

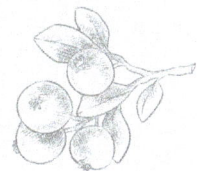

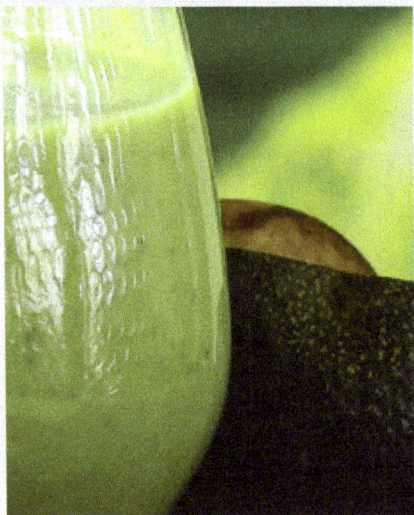

BRAIN-BOOSTING SMOOTHIE

INGREDIENTS

- 4 almonds
- 1 cup coconut water 1 cup packed spinach 1 medium avocado
- 1 cup frozen blueberries 1 tablespoon chia seeds

DIRECTIONS

Mix together all ingredients in the blender. Pulse for 30 seconds on low speed, adjust to high and pulse until smooth. Serve immediately.

NUTRITION FACTS

Calories	277.5kcal
Carbs	30.5g
Protein	5.5g
Fats	33.5g
Fiber	16g
Sugar	9.5g

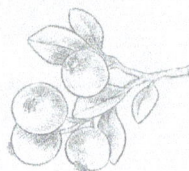

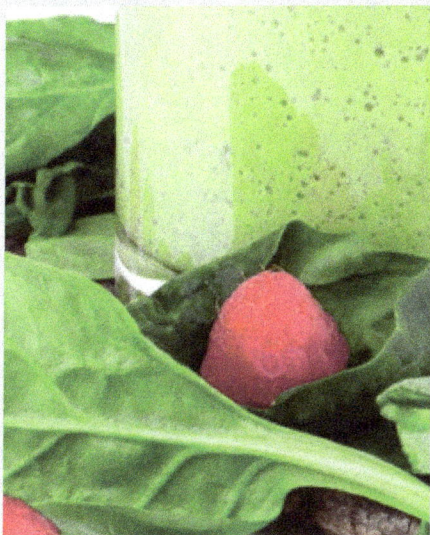

ANTI-INFLAMMATORY SMOOTHIE

INGREDIENTS

- 1 tablespoon hemp seeds 1 cup Greek yogurt
- ½ cup cranberryjuice (optional 2 cups frozen red raspberries
- 1 cup packed spinach
- 1-inch piece fresh ginger root
- 1 to 2 tablespoons of raw honey

DIRECTIONS

Mix together all ingredients in the blender. Pulse for 30 seconds on low speed, adjust to high and pulse until smooth. Serve immediately.

NUTRITION FACTS

Calories	22.5kcal
Carbs	36.5g
Protein	15.5g
Fats	3.8g
Fiber	8.5g
Sugar	25.5g

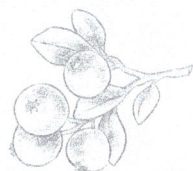

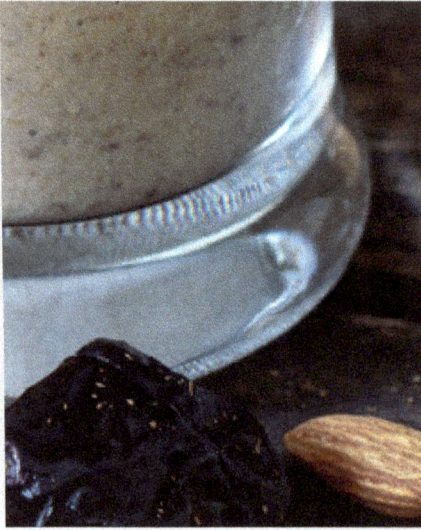

MUSCLE BUILDING SMOOTHIE

INGREDIENTS

- 4 pitted prunes
- 1tablespoon chia or hemp seeds 1 cup Greek yogurt
- 2cups looselypacked kale 2 fresh figs, trimmed
- 1 frozen ripe banana 1 pear

DIRECTIONS

Mix together all ingredients in the blender. Pulse for 30 seconds on low speed, adjust to high and pulse until smooth. Serve immediately.

NUTRITION FACTS

Calories	286kcal
Carbs	55g
Protein	15g
Fats	3.3g
Fiber	9.5g
Sugar	34g

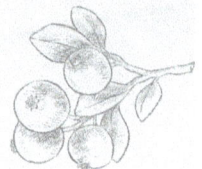

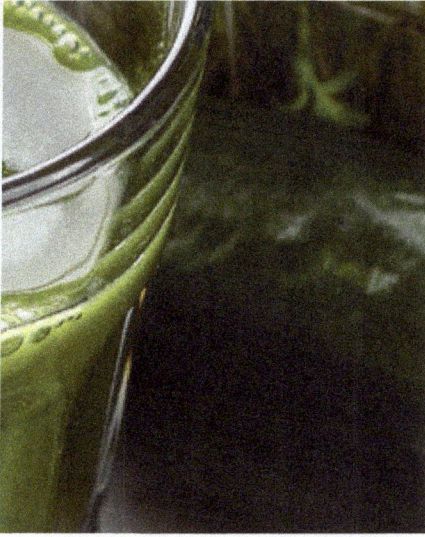

DIGESTIVE ENHANCER SMOOTHIE

INGREDIENTS

- 1 kiwi
- 6 ounces Greek yogurt
- 1 cup loosely packed kale 1 medium cucumber
- 1 medium avocado
- 1 tablespoon of organic lime juice 1 tablespoon of raw honey

DIRECTIONS

Mix together all ingredients in the blender. Pulse for 30 seconds on low speed, adjust to high and pulse until smooth. Serve immediately.

NUTRITION FACTS

Calories	292.5kcal
Carbs	32.5g
Protein	22.5g
Fats	15.5g
Fiber	9g
Sugar	18g

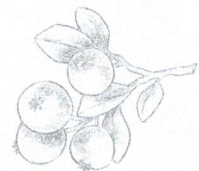

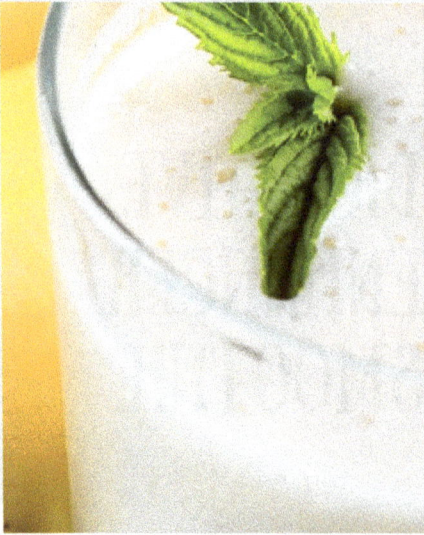

BANANA PEAR SMOOTHIE

INGREDIENTS

- 1 scoop protein powder
  1 pear
- 1 apple (optional)
- ½ cup almond butter
- 2 bananas
- 8 oz Greek yogurt
- ½ teaspoon of
  cinnamon

DIRECTIONS

Mix together all ingredients in the blender. Pulse for 30 seconds on low speed, adjust to high and pulse until smooth. Serve immediately.

NUTRITION FACTS

Calories	265kcal
Carbs	44.5g
Protein	20.5g
Fats	2.5g
Fiber	6.5g
Sugar	25g

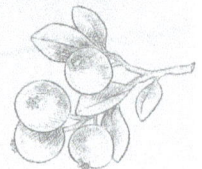

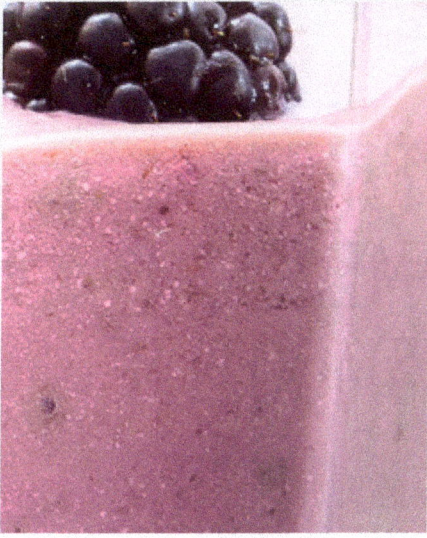

MIXED BERRY SMOOTHIE

INGREDIENTS

- 1scoop why protein powder
- 1 ½ cups frozen blueberry
- ½ cup frozen raspberries
- ½ cup frozen blackberries
- 2tablespoon almond butter
- 1 ½ tablespoons raw honey
- 1 cup unsweetened almond Milk

DIRECTIONS

Mix together all ingredients in the blender. Pulse for 30 seconds on low speed, adjust to high and pulse until smooth. Serve immediately.

NUTRITION FACTS

Calories	295.5kcal
Carbs	40g
Protein	14g
Fats	11g
Fiber	8g
Sugar	23.5g

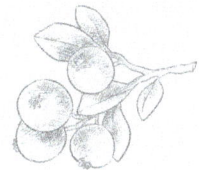

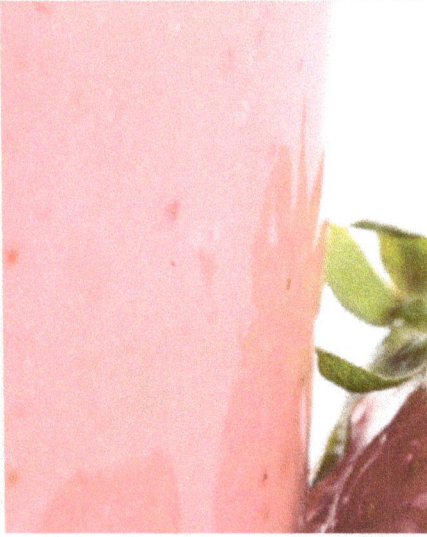

FRUITY MEAL SMOOTHIE

DIRECTIONS

Mix together all ingredients in the blender. Pulse for 30 seconds on low speed, adjust to high and pulse until smooth. Serve immediately.

INGREDIENTS

- 1 banana, peeled
- 1 cup diced mango
- 4 large strawberries
- 1 cup dandelion greens
- 1 tablespoon flax seeds
- 1scoop of protein powder
- 1 cup vanilla almond milk

NUTRITION FACTS

Calories	275.5kcal
Carbs	44g
Protein	4.7g
Fats	44g
Fiber	11.5g
Sugar	28g

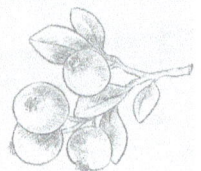

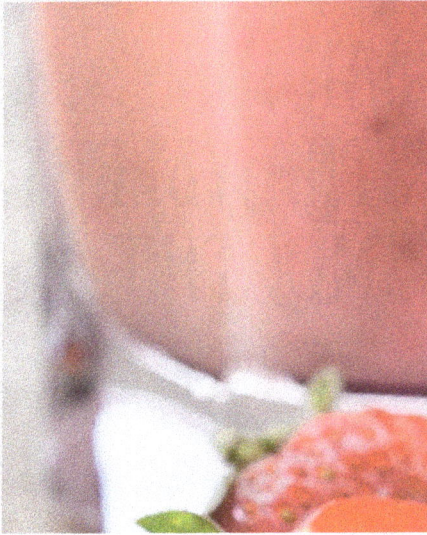

MIXED NUTS & SEEDS SMOOTHIE

INGREDIENTS

- 2 cups frozen strawberries
- 8 almonds
- 1 tablespoon chopped walnuts
- 1 tablespoon flax seed
- 1 tablespoon chia seed
- 1 scoop of protein powder
- 8 ounces of vanilla almond milk

DIRECTIONS

Mix together all ingredients in the blender. Pulse for 30 seconds on low speed, adjust to high and pulse until smooth. Serve immediately.

NUTRITION FACTS

Calories	275.5kcal
Carbs	23g
Protein	17.5g
Fats	13.5g
Fiber	7.5g
Sugar	12.5g

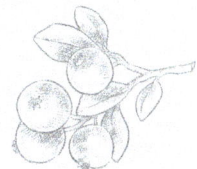

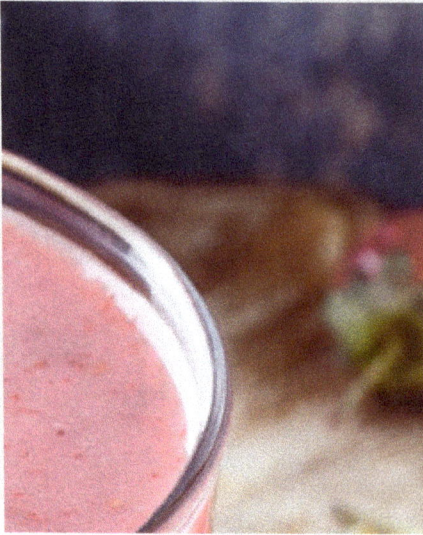

BANANA-STRAWBERRY SMOOTHIE

Preparation time: 5 minutes

Serves: 2

INGREDIENTS

- 1 cup vanilla almond milk
- 1 scoop protein powder
- 1 cup fresh spinach
- 1 banana
- 2 cups frozen strawberries
- 2 tablespoons old-fashioned rolled oats

DIRECTIONS

Mix together all ingredients in the blender. Pulse for 30 seconds on low speed, adjust to high and pulse until smooth. Serve immediately.

NUTRITION FACTS

Calories	286.5kcal
Carbs	47.5g
Protein	17.5g
Fats	4.4g
Fiber	8g
Sugar	26.5g

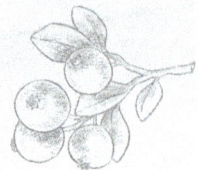

66

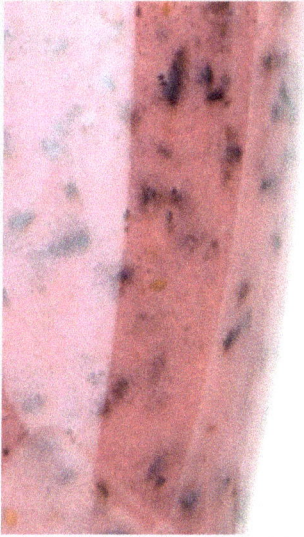

BLUEBERRY KALE SMOOTHIE

Preparation time: 5 minutes

Serves: 2

INGREDIENTS

- 4 ounces Greek yogurt
- 1 scoop soy based protein powder
- 1 cup almond milk
- 20 pine nuts
- 1 cup loosely packed kale
- 2 cups frozen blueberries
- 1 tablespoon maple syrup

DIRECTIONS

Mix together all ingredients in the blender. Pulse for 30 seconds on low speed, adjust to high and pulse until smooth. Serve immediately.

NUTRITION FACTS

Calories	292kcal
Carbs	45.5g
Protein	20.5g
Fats	4.5g
Fiber	6g
Sugar	3.5g

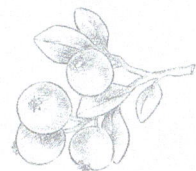

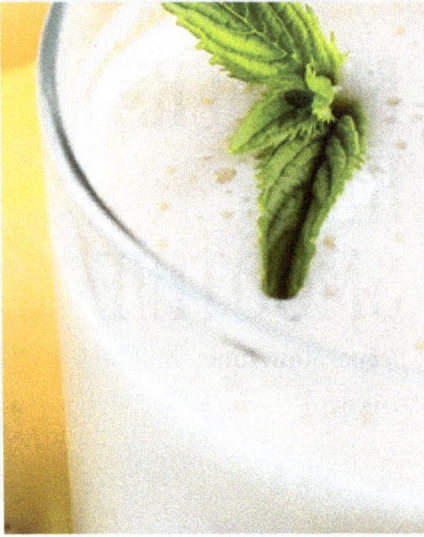

BANANA CARROT SMOOTHIE

Preparation time: 5 minutes

Serves: 2

INGREDIENTS

- ½ cup carrot juice
- 2 bananas
- 1 carrot
- 1 cup sweetened vanilla almond milk
- 1 scoop protein powder
- ½ teaspoon cinnamon

DIRECTIONS

Mix together all ingredients in the blender. Pulse for 30 seconds on low speed, adjust to high and pulse until smooth. Serve immediately.

NUTRITION FACTS

Calories	275kcal
Carbs	38.5g
Protein	28g
Fats	2.5g
Fiber	5.5g
Sugar	18g

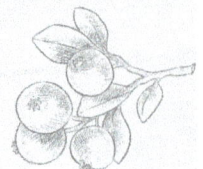

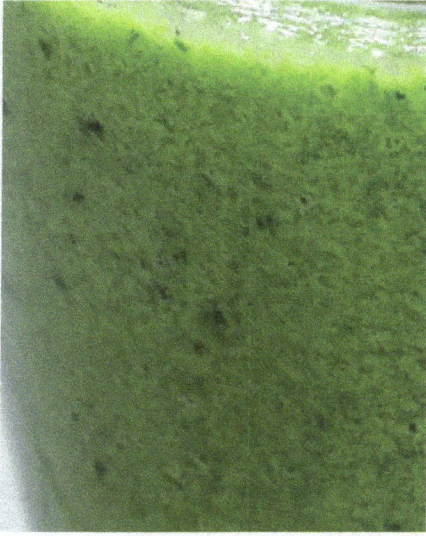

APPLE COCONUT SMOOTHI

Preparation time: 5 minutes

Serves: 2

INGREDIENTS

- 6 ounces Greek yogurt
- ½ cup shredded coconut meat
- ¼ cup almonds
- ½ teaspoon cinnamon
- 2 apples
- 1 scoop protein powder
- 1 tablespoon flax seeds

DIRECTIONS

Mix together all ingredients in the blender. Pulse for 30 seconds on low speed, adjust to high and pulse until smooth. Serve immediately.

NUTRITION FACTS

Calories	298kcal
Carbs	34.5g
Protein	23.5g
Fats	10g
Fiber	8.5g
Sugar	23g

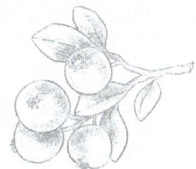

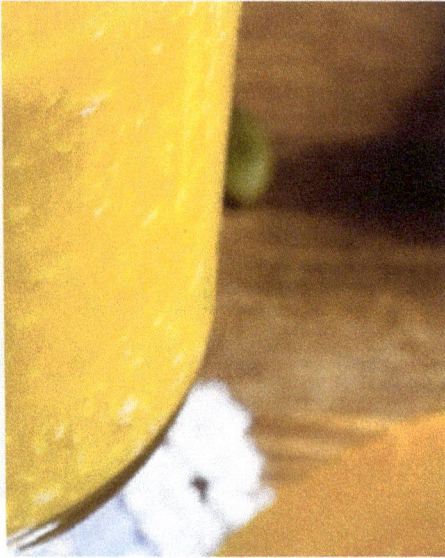

PUMPKIN PROTEIN SMOOTHIE

Preparation time: 5 minutes

Serves: 2

INGREDIENTS

- 1 cup Greekyogurt
- 1cup unsaltedcanned pumpkin
- 1 ½ scoop protein powder
- 2 tablespoons cashew nuts
- 1 cup loosely packed kale
- 1 tablespoon raw honey
- 1 pinch of ground nutmeg

DIRECTIONS

Mix together all ingredients in the blender. Pulse for 30 seconds on low speed, adjust to high and pulse until smooth. Serve immediately.

NUTRITION FACTS

Calories	280kcal
Carbs	21.5g
Protein	34.5g
Fats	7.5g
Fiber	5.5g
Sugar	9g

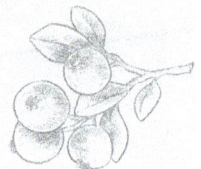

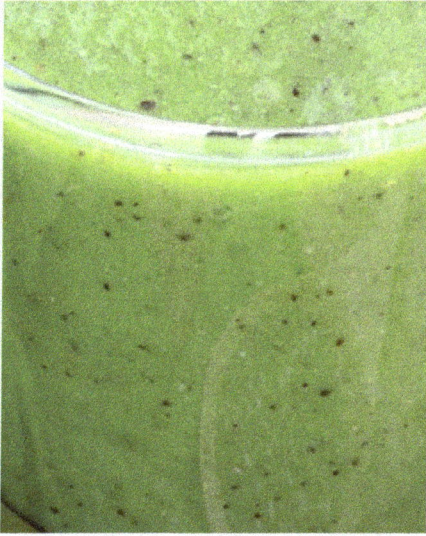

GRAPE SPINACH SMOOTHIE

Preparation time: 5 minutes

Serves: 2

INGREDIENTS

- 2 cups seedless frozen green grapes
- 2 cups of spinach
- ½ cup coconut water
- 1 cup Greek yogurt
- 2 tablespoons chia seeds
- 1 tablespoon of raw honey

DIRECTIONS

Mix together all ingredients in the blender. Pulse for 30 seconds on low speed, adjust to high and pulse until smooth. Serve immediately.

NUTRITION FACTS

Calories	290kcal
Carbs	45.5g
Protein	16.5g
Fats	5.5g
Fiber	7.5g
Sugar	27.5g

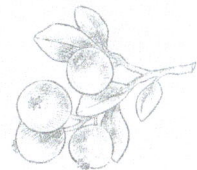

Index

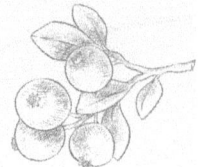

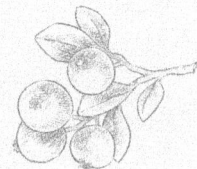

About the Book

Our book offers a harmonious blend of recipes tailored for various health needs. Whether managing diabetes, promoting gut health, aiming for weight loss, seeking longevity, or navigating diseases such as cancer, we've crafted a range of nutrient-packed smoothies to support your journey.

Indulge in vibrant flavors and wholesome ingredients that not only tantalize your taste buds but also nourish your body. From refreshing citrus concoctions to antioxidant-rich berry blends, each sip is a step towards a healthier you.

Explore specialized diets such as Keto and Atkins with dedicated sections in our book. ' Healthy Smoothies' empowers you to enjoy delicious smoothies while staying true to your dietary preferences.

Join the chorus of health enthusiasts and let 'Healthy Smoothies' be your guide to a vibrant and energized lifestyle. Blend, sip, and thrive with every recipe!"

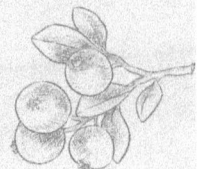

About the Authors

Introducing Dr. Kelafo and Dr. Shallaywa Collie, a dynamic husband-and-wife duo whose passion for exploring cuisines and promoting healthy eating has taken the culinary world by storm. Both accomplished doctors, renowned international authors, avid travelers, and sought-after motivational speakers and life coaches, they bring a unique blend of expertise and enthusiasm to their latest project—a revolutionary recipe book designed to inspire and empower readers to embrace a healthier lifestyle through delicious, nutritious recipes.

With a wealth of experience in medicine and a deep understanding of the importance of nutrition in overall well-being, Doctors Collie have meticulously crafted a collection of recipes that not only tantalize the taste buds but also nourish the body and mind. From vibrant salads bursting with fresh, seasonal ingredients to velvety smoothies packed with antioxidants and vitality-boosting nutrients; each dish in their recipe book is a testament to their commitment to wholesome eating. Drawing inspiration from their travels around the globe, their recipes are infused with diverse flavors and culinary techniques, ensuring that every meal is a celebration of culinary artistry and healthful living.

This book aims to empower readers to make informed choices about their health while savoring the joys of cooking and sharing wholesome meals with loved ones. Whether you're craving a comforting bowl of soup on a chilly evening or a refreshing smoothie too, here's to kickstarting your day!

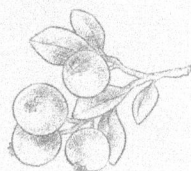

www.ingramcontent.com/pod-product-compliance
Lightning Source LLC
Chambersburg PA
CBHW070907280326
41934CB00008B/1612